MID-LIFE CRISIS MAN

A Man's Guide to Surviving Middle Age

By Henri (Renoir) Rennie

Cartoons by Angus Gardner

Dear Paige and Jack

Thank you for all your support and help! Henri
xx

Mid-Life Crisis MANagement
Copyright © 2016 Henri 'Renoir' Rennie
All rights reserved.

ISBN: 978-0-9946174-8-4

Published by Meredian Pictures & Words 2016
Angels Beach, Australia

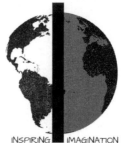

MEREDIAN
PICTURES & WORDS

INSPIRING IMAGINATION

> "Every man desires to live long;
> but no man wishes to be old."
> *- Jonathon Swift*
> British satirist and poet 1667 - 1745

For Matt who suggested it
and Meredith who supported and encouraged it.

With thanks to Angus
for illustrating it.

CONTENTS

.o0o.

About the Author

Who is Henri Rennie, anyway?

I'm not a doctor. Or a psychologist. Or any sort of professional New Age therapist, though I've studied a fair bit. I'm a bloke who asks questions, and writes down the answers in a way that other blokes will understand.

For a long time I've been interested in health and healing. I've done First Aid and Lifesaving Certificates, training in Occupational Health & Safety, a Certificate in Reiki and been trained as a Nutrition Advisor at the Sanoviv Medical Institute in Baja California.

I've turned my hand at a lot of jobs over the years. At various times I've been an actor, a barman, a journo, and coached a (pretty ordinary) soccer team. I've sung in a 70's suburban rock band, and been a greenkeeper, a plumber's mate, a Public Servant, a security guard, even a vacuum cleaner salesman.

I've worked in offices and pubs, on building sites and on the road, in colleges and in jail.

Along the way I've probably eaten and drunk more than I should have, and exercised less than was good for me. I've had what feels like a filing cabinet full of my own health issues. Lots of the common ones – broken legs, kidney stones, asthma and pneumonia, heart attack, and some less common – busted spine, three types of arthritis all at once, some of my guts removed.

Family, friends and acquaintances have been through a bunch of stuff too. Some survived, others didn't.

But I've been lucky – I've survived, and learned as I went along.

These days I travel quite a bit, talking to people and trying to learn stuff as I go. Mostly I write.

I've learned a lot of facts, looked at statistics, gathered some opinions and formed some of my own. And now I'm sharing that with you.

Sometimes I'm known as 'Renoir' when I'm writing fiction, or drawing cartoons.

But this is another part of me. This part wants to do more than make people laugh. This part sees blokes suffering, often (not always) in silence and wants to do something to help. The *Quiet Word* books are my way of trying to do that.

Blokes don't often talk face to face – we talk better shoulder to shoulder. That's why we have better conversations in the car or standing at the bar than over the dinner table.

Even then, there's a lot we don't talk much about out loud, even to our mates. Like our health. Think of this book as a quiet word – a quiet word that might save your life.

.o0o.

FOREWORD

It is not uncommon for middle aged men to ignore and neglect their health. This lack of attention often means that men present with advanced disease which could have been identified and managed earlier if medical attention had been sought.

Improved physical and mental condition with advancing age is a clear benefit for men who pay attention to their health care needs.

This book identifies the key issues in men's health that should be addressed if one is seeking an optimal quality of life with advancing age.

I strongly recommend that men read and take notice of its messages.

Professor Darrell Crawford MD FRACP
Head of The School of Medicine, University of Queensland
Director of Research, Gallipoli Medical Research Foundation
Practising Gastroenterologist

INTRODUCTION – Why This Book?

I was standing in the bar having a chat with my old friend Matt. We'd had a couple of drinks, so the conversation had taken a serious turn.

Not, well, you know, Deep And Meaningful – we were still a few drinks short of that. But we had moved on to talking about more than cars and football.

Specifically, we were discussing how long we'd known each other: how our lives had changed, how we'd changed, what might be on the horizon.

"It worries me," said Matt. "Three blokes I know, they all lost it when they got into their mid-forties or so. One committed suicide. One wrapped his car round a tree – might as well call it suicide from what I can make out. One got shot and killed by the police when he went nuts and attacked them! What's the story with that?"

We're blokes. We're not good at talking about our health – physical or mental. We make jokes about our own and others' "mid-life crises". We tell caustic and cautionary tales about women's "change of life".

It takes the sting out of it. Easier than admitting to anyone, including ourselves, that there's a problem. Or even just that we're worried there *might* be a problem.

But really – what's the point of spending forty-odd years making money, or "making a life", then spending the rest of that life spending that money on doctors just to stay alive?

I realised that like Matt I'm in the age range where the body goes through some important changes. Some blokes barely notice, others have a tough time and don't understand why. Most of us don't talk about it.

"What's the story with that?" he asked, and I wondered.

I've read a lot, and talked with (more importantly *listened* to) a lot of people who are experts in their fields. I've tried to avoid a lot of the jargon and technical terms that medical people and therapists like to throw about. When I've had to use their language to explain something, I've tried to break it down into terms I'd understand if I was still standing in the bar with Matt.

You can read from cover to cover, or dip into whatever you think might be relevant to you. That's what chapter headings and the Index are for.

Look out for the **Simply put:** boxes. They're where I've stripped out the detail and given you stuff in a nutshell.

"What's the story with that?" he asked.

Here's what I've found out...

.o0o.

1 TELL ME ABOUT THIS "CHANGE" THING…

Okay, first things first. Yes, it's real.

It might be hard to define, more so for some blokes than others. It might be less obvious than the changes many women go through. It might not get talked about or written about a lot, but it is DEFINITELY real.

The Change. Mid-life crisis. Male menopause. Andropause. The 48 Crash. Multiple names and even more potential symptoms. You might cop it bad, or you may barely notice any change at all.

If you're one of the lucky ones, that's great and I'm happy for you. If you're not (and you're not just kidding yourself about that) then I figure it's better that *you* take charge of *it* than it takes charge of you.

And there are three keys to doing that.

1. Understanding what is, or might be happening to you.
2. Admitting it – even to yourself.
3. Then doing something about it. Read on!

The 'doing' bit is the big step. I'll get into some practical options later, some of which I hope will do you some good. But first, I want to look at some info. It's hard to win a fight when you know nothing about who or what you're up against.

1.1 It's not a quick change

Despite what Suzi Quatro sang, the "48 Crash" does not strike 'like a lightning flash'.

One of the big differences between what happens to blokes and what happens to women is that for many of the ladies it's sudden. One month everything is happening the same way it's done since they were teenagers – the next month it's not, and they're getting hot flushes and other unpleasant surprises. (Okay, it's not that simple and certainly not the same for every woman either, but you get the idea.)

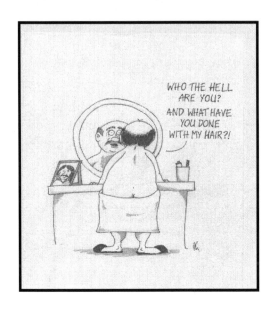

For blokes it's usually a lot more gradual, happening progressively over years from around the age of thirty. And the thing about gradual change is that we tend not to notice it until it passes a certain point, or until something 'external' causes us to notice it.

It's like driving over a long distance in one long session at the wheel. You stop being particularly aware of your speed – whether you've been gradually speeding up or slowing down. Then you glance down at the speedo and go "Jeez – when did I get up to 140 clicks?" or "Strewth – I'm only doing 60, I must be dozing off!" Or suddenly another car or truck whizzes past you, or their tail lights loom in front of you a whole lot quicker than you expected. It's only then you take notice and realise you're not doing the speed you used to be doing.

"I have the body of an 18-year-old.
I keep it in the fridge."

- Spike Milligan

Irish author, poet and comedian 1918 - 2002

Your body is made up of between five and ten *trillion* cells. Almost all of them have a limited life span. (The exceptions are in your brain. The neurons you grow in childhood are pretty much all you get.) They die and get replaced every few days or every few weeks (depending on where they are – the skin, for example, has a really rapid 'turnover'). When that replacement process doesn't work as well as it should, or as well as it used to, the body starts to degenerate. It might show up as chronic conditions like heart disease, or cancer, or diabetes, or we might just call it 'ageing'.

The ageing process is controllable. There are still things that you can do to slow down the "rate of decay". Statistically, the odds are you'll live to at least 70 whether you like it or not. So you may as well do whatever you can to *like* it, eh?

Simply put: getting older happens. It doesn't

have to make a mess of you, or your life.

1.2 It's never too early, or too late

You might be reading this thinking "Lucky I'm too young for any of this to matter to me yet – I'm years away from middle age!" Sorry mate, but you're wrong.

The earlier you start looking after yourself, the easier the job can be long term. (Lying in a cardiac ward writing notes for this book, I wished I'd realised that a few decades ago!)

Imagine if when you turned seventeen you were given a new car. Brand new, top of the range, in perfect condition – a car that had plenty of power, responsive handling, and comfort. You could accessorise it or hot it up as much or as little as you like. Just one catch: you're told it's the only car you can ever have. *Ever*. No trade-ins, no updated models.

How well do you reckon that car would be looked after? Something shows signs of wear, it'd get fixed or replaced real quick! Regular servicing? Too right! Save a few bucks using dodgy oil or the wrong fuel because it's cheaper? I don't think so. Damaged in an accident? Don't just patch it up, get a proper repair job done.

For most of us, the body we get once puberty has finished working us over is that car. You can work on it, hot it up, build it up or even pretty it up, but it's as good as it will be without enhancement.

Unfortunately a lot of us don't take the same sort of care with our bodies as we do with our replaced-every-few-years cars. We put in any sort of junk as fuel. Chuck in all sorts of additives we know aren't good for us. Avoid doctors because they'll only give you bad news anyway and it really doesn't feel too bad. Take knocks and bumps on the sports ground but play on anyway: "It'll be right, mate."

And we wonder why we wake up full of aches and pains one day, when our hair's going grey or falling out, our chest seems to have slipped down to our belly and running up the stairs turns on funny little twinkling lights in front of our eyes.

The earlier in life you start doing positive stuff, the more effective it's likely to be, but it's never too late to do something.

"Man is born to live, not prepare for life."

- Boris Pasternak

Russian novelist, author of 'Doctor Zhivago' 1890 - 1960

I read a quote from a competitive figure skater recently: "As you grow older if you don't move you won't move." The skater in question is 88 years old.

Even more extreme is the English bloke who's reckoned to be "the world's fittest pensioner".

Charles Eugster is his name. He's a retired dentist, now living in Switzerland. He'd lived a pretty ordinary life, not knocking himself about too badly but not looking after himself especially well either. As he tells it, "I looked in the mirror one morning and didn't like what I saw."

He started running and rowing. All this happened when he was 85.

He decided after a while that his muscles needed work, so at 87 he took up bodybuilding.

Charles isn't stupid. He wears a heart monitor when he's working out, and will stop if he finds he's overdoing it. But at 94 he's a World Masters rowing champion, still lifting weights that would challenge blokes half his age, and training for the 1000 metre run.

"This training is my job for life," he said in an interview. "If I don't keep exercising I'm dead – this is keeping me alive."

Becoming a gym junkie might not appeal to you. I can sympathise. I can push myself into spending a bit of time at the gym, but it isn't something I'm driven to do every day. The point is though that you're never too old to make some changes for the better, even if they're a challenge. Just do it carefully and sensibly.

"When they tell me I'm too old to do something, I attempt it immediately."

- Pablo Picasso

Spanish artist 1881 - 1973

Sometimes those changes might not produce much in the way of obvious results. If you're not hugely overweight then changing flab back into muscle might not show up much on the bathroom scales. (The numbers may even look worse – muscle is heavier than fat.) Your hair's not likely to grow back. You might not feel that the walk to and from the corner store is getting much quicker or easier. But the important thing is that it's not getting worse.

The important thing is that if you aren't doing anything, you *will* eventually notice the difference. Even in your twenties the signs are there. Slowly if you're lucky, but surely, you'll start to see them. The paunch is getting bigger. The skin is getting greyer. The breathing is getting tougher when you do try to exert yourself walking, running, climbing or whatever.

> **Simply put:** whatever age you are, taking action
> may not always actually make you feel much better,
> but it will stop you feeling worse.

If you've already hit middle age and you're feeling it, there are still things you can do to stop things from getting worse. And there are definitely some things that you *can* improve.

Knowledge is power, so I've heard. But it's a two-step process. Any knowledge is really only powerful when you actually apply it.

"Every man is the architect of his own fate."

- Appius Claudius

Roman statesman @300 B.C.

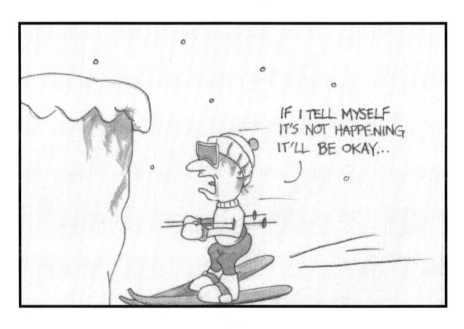

I'll tell you what I've learned about 'male menopause' and 'mid-life crisis' in blokes – causes, symptoms, and related conditions. And I'll explain what I can about various things that might be helpful for

16

you. But for that information to really be useful, then *you* have to do something with it.

So let's start building the knowledge. Let's really define what it is we're talking about.

.o0o.

2 WHAT EXACTLY IS IT?

I'll start with a couple of definitions so you know what I'm on about.

'Menopause' is a medical term. It refers to a specific physical change that happens in the body. It has to do with the production of hormones, and what happens when there are less of them than there used to be. I'll go into more detail about that in a minute.

The expression 'mid-life crisis' is a bit more vague. It's thought of as a psychological thing: restlessness of spirit, dissatisfaction, 'irrational' decisions, anxiety – at its worst depression that can go as far as suicide.

The two really go together. A lot of what goes on in your mind is directly related to what's going on in your body, whether it's obvious or not. It's chemistry, and it's why drugs like anti-depressants work. It's also why recreational drugs (legal or otherwise) have the effects that they do in cheering you up or bringing you down.

2.1 Defining 'male menopause'

There are a number of doctors who won't actually use the term "male menopause" even though they admit the reality of what's happening in a man's body. They might call it 'andropause', although that term isn't recognised by the World Health Organisation. Another term used is 'late-onset hypogonadism' – a mouthful that officially translates as 'a deficiency in male hormone levels beyond expected levels in an ageing man'.

The closest to a plain English term that I could find is 'testosterone deficiency'. That's getting there, if a bit misleading. Like I said earlier, as blokes get older we produce less testosterone. We still produce the stuff, sometimes even into our seventies and beyond, just a smaller amount each month. The UK's National Health Service (NHS) suggests the average rate of decline is one to two percent every year, usually starting somewhere between the ages of 30 and 40.

One thing that can make male menopause more evident for some blokes is if they produce a below-average amount of testosterone to begin with. That doesn't necessarily mean they've been impotent. Different guys simply produce different amounts – some more than others – and it's common sense that if you start with lower numbers then as production naturally decreases you'll more quickly be 'below expected levels'.

Many older men will have testosterone levels similar to those of men in their thirties. Perhaps about one in 200 men under 60 and one in 10 men over 60 have 'abnormally' low testosterone levels (i.e. significantly below the average for their age).

"Youth is immortal, 'tis only the elderly that grow old!"

- Herman Melville

U.S. author 1819 - 1891

It's not just testosterone that's affected. There are chemicals called anabolic hormones. It means they contribute to tissue growth. You might have heard or read of some like DHEA (dehydroepianandrosterone), MGF (mechano growth factor) and IGF-1 (insulin-like growth factor 1) in the sports pages. Some of them have a specific role to play in muscle development.

Production of these Human Growth Hormones – the drug-cheating athlete's friend – tapers off dramatically as we age. That makes sense when you think about it – if he spent his whole life growing at the rate that he grew as a kid the average bloke would be at least eighteen foot tall and eight foot wide by his eightieth birthday.

Testosterone and hormone production are connected to a lot more than just sex drive. There are lots of other chemical reactions in the body that are affected. I'll get into detail in the next chapters, but effects can include fatigue, muscle weakness, increased sweating, mood swings, and finding it harder to concentrate.

It becomes a "medical condition" when the rate of decline is significantly higher than the average rate, and/or when the average amount of testosterone in the body is consistently well below the average amount for a man of that age. That's a doctor's opinion. If you're the bloke in question, though, you're not likely to know that average figure or even care about it. What matters to you is the realisation that in some way you're not the bloke you used to be.

The Mayo Clinic website talks about "the myth of male menopause" and says its effects "aren't necessarily clear". Some doctors may say similar things to you. But there's plenty of evidence that says otherwise, as you'll see in the coming pages.

Others, like Matty Silver, a 'Sexual Health Therapist' writing in the Sydney Morning Herald, reckon many of the symptoms "are a normal part of ageing." Well, menopause in women is a normal part of ageing, and it gets taken, and treated, seriously. Why shouldn't that be the case for us, when **we** know and admit there's a problem?

Simply put: male menopause is when the level of hormones in a bloke's body is consistently below a point where the physical state of the body changes.

2.2 Defining 'mid-life crisis'

The UK's National Health Service calls male 'mid-life crisis' a "controversial syndrome that (some) health experts think is related to the brain or hormonal changes", with symptoms that are anxiety or stress based. See above. The two go together.

It's tough to define, but you know it when you're in it. Blokes going through it often use words such as "aimless", "confused" and "lost." It can mean questioning things in which they once believed – their marriage, work, and/or friendships. In the book *Flyfishing through the Midlife Crisis*, the New York Times executive editor Howell Raines describes this feeling as "disappointment and restlessness that tiptoe in on little cat feet."

That's more like a list of symptoms than a real definition. Depression can be associated with it, and might be a result of it, but it isn't the same thing.

The key for me is in the term 'mid-life'. Somewhere between 40 and 45, a lot of us suddenly realise we're about half way through the lifespan we reckon we might reasonably expect.

But it isn't so much an exact age as is it a state of mind. I read about a bloke who declared himself "middle-aged" at 36. He said that he got on a bus and realised that half the people he could see were older than him and half younger. He thus concluded that he was middle-aged, and immediately had himself convinced that his life was half over.

"Old age is the most unexpected of all things that happen to a man."

- Leon Trotsky

Russian revolutionary 1879 - 1940

It's also about what that realization means to you. How you react to it.

It's like the half time break, when the coach gets the team together and looks at what's been achieved so far. The score doesn't necessarily matter. Some coaches will find the positives, emphasise them and encourage the boys. Other coaches won't be pleased whatever the lead, and will point out every single mistake. It might inspire the boys to perform better, but it might just make matters worse by knocking out whatever self-confidence they had left.

That's where the crisis is: focusing on the negatives. We're the coach inside our own head and if all we hear is criticism, that's what we'll respond to.

> **Simply put:** the mid-life crisis is when a bloke decides to himself that he's hit 'middle age', starts asking himself some questions about his life, and doesn't like the answers.

2.3 It's not the same as women get.

A lot of blokes don't know much about menopause or 'change of life' in women. A lot don't really want to, but I reckon it's handy information if there's a woman, or women in your life that you care about. This won't help you to Understand Women, but it will give you an idea of what they might be going through.

Dr. Raymond Burnett is an obstetrician from Chicago. His book *"Menopause – All Your Questions Answered"* is packed with good information, but he writes like a doctor. I've tried to make it a bit easier for the average bloke to follow.

Menopause in a woman is really a single point in time. If you did all the right medical tests you could just about actually mark it on a graph.

Girls are born with all their eggs already formed – about 700,000 of them. They've lost maybe half of those by the time they hit puberty, after which a batch of them start to mature in her ovaries every month. That monthly cycle of egg-maturing is when the hormone estrogen is getting produced in large quantities. The great majority of that batch of maturing eggs die off – the remaining mature one travels from the ovary to the uterus and is that one that gets fertilised if the timing is right. If that doesn't happen the egg is lost during her period.

Eventually the ovaries pretty much run out of eggs. That's the point at which her body's need for a regular period stops. That's "menopause". It's also the point when the production of estrogen drops way down and a lot of other chemical effects start to happen – producing a lot of the stuff that gets lumped together as "change of life".

Simply put: menopause in women has an identifiable starting point, although the effects might sometimes continue to be felt and seen for a long time afterwards.

Blokes differ right from the start. We're born with no sperm. Zero. Puberty is when we start producing it, together with a bunch of hormones that make us what we are. Production hits peak early, then tapers off gradually.

In the late teens and early twenties production hits its highest levels, but it continues for decades. A bloke in his seventies isn't likely to be producing sperm (and associated body chemicals) like he did when he was seventeen. Unlike a woman of the same age though he is still generating hormones.

It's not something that's been extensively researched, but since 2003 there's been evidence presented that hormone production in men rises and falls in twenty to thirty day cycles, paralleling the maturation of eggs in women.

If you were among the many people who took an interest in biorhythms when they were an "in thing" back in the 1970's, those numbers might be familiar.

Although biorhythms have supposedly been discredited as 'pseudoscience' (for example in a 1981 report done by NASA) due to some very dodgy testing of the theory, scientists are happy to accept the concept of chronobiology. That's the technical name for studying periodic cyclic phenomena in living beings. So there is recognition that some biological things happen to a rhythm or cycle.

One of the accepted examples of such a phenomenon is the 28-day human menstrual cycle. Given the number of elements of the body's functions that are affected by hormones – not just the obvious sex-related ones - I don't reckon it's unreasonable to suggest that we peak and trough across a month. Such a rhythm wouldn't necessarily begin on the day of birth. Before detachment from the placenta, the unborn baby's internal functions are already responding to its mother's body chemistry.

So while further research might actually reveal a 23- or 25- or 28-day biological cycle for blokes, actually pinning down the day it starts (and thus making accurate predictions about what's to come) seems further away.

Suffice to say that while the cycle of hormone production may continue for many years, the 'peak production points' get gradually lower. So there are simply lesser quantities of testosterone, DHEA, growth hormones etc. available for the body to work with. At some point those quantities, even at the peak of production, drop below the level required for some bodily functions to work.

If you drew it as a really simplified graph it might look like this:

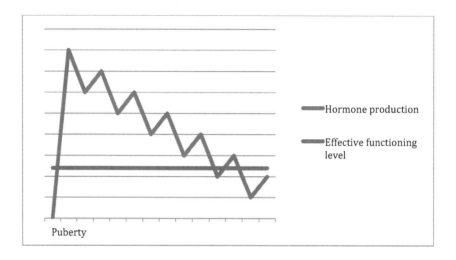

Once you're staying below that red line, that's male menopause.

Simply put: although there are obvious physical differences, it's clear that age brings change to male bodies as much as females'.

.o0o.

3 HOW IT MIGHT AFFECT YOUR BODY

There are a number of physical symptoms of 'mid-life'. Where it gets confusing is that while there are several things that can be linked directly to chemical changes connected to lower levels of hormones in the body, some of those things can also be caused by other factors. Some of them can be the result of a build-up of years of abuse or neglect – but the 'ageing process' can be what makes them suddenly obvious, or harder to ignore.

According to a 2008 study by the Australian Institute of Health & Welfare, the ten leading causes of death for Aussie men were:

1 Coronary heart disease	18.5%
2 Lung cancer	7%
3 Stroke	6.9%
4 Other heart diseases	4.8%
5 Prostate cancer	4.4%
6 Chronic Obstructive Pulmonary Disease	4.2%
7 Bowel cancer	3.5%
8 Unknown primary site cancers	2.7%
9 Diabetes	2.6%
10 Suicide	2.5%

(You can add skin cancer onto that list - in the last few years it's become increasingly obvious that years of sun-worshipping are catching up with us.)

Ageing has a part to play in most if not all of them. Sometimes it's just wear and tear, or lack of proper maintenance. And sometimes the chemical changes in your body that come with 'mid-life' can be either triggers or contributing factors.

The website of the National Health Service (NHS) in the UK lists the most common physical symptoms of male menopause as:

- hot flushes (it's more complicated than that – see below)
- excessive sweating
- dry and/or thin skin
- loss of muscle mass
- fat redistribution
- erectile dysfunction
- loss of sex drive.

That last one could be as much psychological as physical. I'll give it some attention a bit later, I promise.

There are a couple of other recognised effects too:

- decrease in bone density
- increased risk of cardiovascular disease
- higher blood pressure.

Like I said, any or all of these can be caused by age changing your body chemistry, or by other wear and tear you've gone through, or a combination of both.

Not all of them are potentially fatal, although some certainly are. But any and all of them can really mess with your quality of life, as anyone suffering knows far too well. A long slow deterioration can make death feel like a less daunting prospect than it used to be.

> ## "We are living too short, and dying too long."
> *- Dr. Myron Wentz*
> Einstein Award-winning biochemist

3.1 The heat is on

The NHS' description of 'hot flushes' is misleading, I reckon. For one thing, it makes it easy to dismiss the symptom, or try to ignore it "cos it's a womens' thing".

More importantly, it overlooks the underlying cause of 'hot flushes' – what's going on with your blood.

Here's a bit of body chemistry that you might not have known. You've got estrogen in your body, just like a woman does. And the funny thing is, it's actually made by your body converting a small percentage of your testosterone. That's okay – it's normal, and has an important role to play in day-to-day life. In fact, it's not unusual for a post-menopausal woman to have less estrogen in her body than a bloke of the same age.

That small amount of estrogen does a lot of useful things. One of those is helping to drive a part of your brain called the hypothalamus. When the level of estrogen falls, the hypothalamus is adversely affected. As the hypothalamus regulates your body temperature, the decrease in estrogen causes the brain to incorrectly detect too much body heat.

As a natural reaction to this, it seems the brain releases hormones like serotonin that are supposed to help lower body heat. But in fact what happens is that they cause the heart rate to rise and blood vessels to dilate in order to allow more blood to flow through and dissipate the heat.

The increased blood flow causes the body to produce its natural cooling method - sweat. This series of events is what creates that heated, sweaty feeling which people who don't suffer from it dismiss as something of a joke.

> **Simply put:** a 'hot flush' is when a chemical in your brain makes your body think that it's overheated, even when it isn't, and reacts in a way that makes you feel like it really is hot.

A really good reason not to ignore this particular symptom is that a particular type of cancer – a tumour affecting the endocrine system that secretes a large amount of serotonin, can cause exactly the same sort of hot flushes.

I'm not saying this to panic you. Endocrine tumour is an uncommon form of cancer. But it's out there, and if you've suddenly started getting the sweats for no apparent reason, and no other obvious symptoms, it's a good thing to be able to cross off the list of possible causes. And you can't do that if you don't talk to someone and get some tests done.

> **Simply put:** hot flushes and increased sweating don't necessarily mean there's something "wrong" with a bloke, but they can be warning signs.

3.2 Skin – It's a wrap

Your skin does more than just stop all the wobbly bits from falling out as you walk down the street.

It's your biggest organ, accounting for about 16% of your weight. It replaces itself every 27 days, so in the space of a year you shed about 500g of dead skin. And it does a bunch of important stuff:

- It acts as a barrier to keep microorganisms and toxic chemicals from having easy access to your innards.

- It lets some fluids in and keeps other out to ensure your survival.

- It helps maintain your body temperature.

- It's the key component of your sense of touch.

Here's a thing: your skin is the last organ to get nourishment from the body, and it's the first to show signs of nutritional problems, chemical imbalance, illness and in particular ageing.

The natural ageing process of the skin is a continuous thing that normally begins in our mid-20s, although the signs may not be visible for decades.

The top layer of skin (the epidermis) slows down its cell production. The very top surface layer dries out more, and with the dehydration you're left with cells that are mostly protein (keratin – the stuff that's in your hair and fingernails) and little or no moisture. When that happens the skin can get dry and flaky, even powdery. A bit like all-over dandruff.

At that layer you also start to have less "Langerhans cells". These useful little blokes are a type of immune cell that do a lot of that bacteria and toxin fighting I mentioned earlier. So when they decrease you're more likely to pick up infections and skin diseases.

The epidermis is also home to pigment cells that give your skin its colour. The number of these cells decreases with age, but those that are left increase in size. That means the ageing skin appears thinner and paler. Large pigmented spots (you might hear them called called age spots, liver spots, or lentigos) may appear in areas of the skin that cop a lot of sun.

At the next layer down (the dermis) collagen and elastin production slows. Those are the substances that enable skin to snap back into place, so as you age it has a bit less spring. Ultimately, that means wrinkles and sagging.

This is the layer where your skin produces the oils that keep it naturally moist, and as you age the tiny glands responsible for this get less efficient. So your skin dehydrates and is more easily damaged by harsh soaps and disinfectants. Stuff that 'cleans' you by stripping the oils and moisture out of your skin along with the dirt is doing more harm than good.

The dermis is also where the skin's blood vessels sit. They gradually get fewer, and weaker. So the skin loses its "glow". Worse, it suffers and shows damage much more easily – stuff like bruising, purpura (bleeding under the skin) or cherry angioma (a small, bright red skin growth, sometimes a lump, made up of blood vessels).

At the bottom is the subcutaneous layer. It's mostly fat. It's the insulation layer, both for temperature and shock. Sadly, as we age that's one place where fat levels decline so the skin sags and hangs looser than it used to. Add that to what I said about the dermis, and there's where your wrinkles come from.

If all of that isn't enough, there are a number of external factors that often act together with the normal ageing process to prematurely age our skin.

The most obvious is sun exposure. Ultraviolet radiation damages collagen and elastin, so that wrinkled leathery look happens sooner rather than later. Add in freckles, age spots, spider veins, actinic keratoses (thick, rough, reddish patches of skin that resemble warts), and worst of all, skin cancer and you get the picture: too much sun is a Bad Thing.

Remember, it doesn't have to be hot and blazing to affect the skin. Those are just the days when it's obvious – sunburn is the warning flag that goes up too late. Even on a cool cloudy day you're getting hit by a dose of solar radiation and it all adds up.

Other external factors that prematurely age our skin are:

> - repetitive facial expressions (laughter and frown lines),
>
> - gravity (jowls happen, noses droop and earlobes get bigger),
>
> - sleeping positions (lines from nightly pressure on the same part of the face),
>
> - smoking (chemical reactions dry and yellow the skin).

Another skin-related thing that can hit in middle age is an unsightly growth on the end of your nose. You know the thing I mean – it looks like the end of a sausage when you're cooking it and the meat squeezes out of the casing.

W.C. Fields called it his 'gin blossom', but its real name is *rhinophyma* (which just means 'nose growth'). It happens when skin cells, often the oil-producing ones, on the end of the nose go into overdrive.

It swells into a red bulb shape, the pores get big, and the outer layer of skin gradually gets thick and rough, even waxy.

For years the condition was blamed on long-term alcohol abuse. If you're a sufferer, that's probably what you've been accused of by people who don't know any better. But the truth is, while heavy drinking can aggravate matters, it's not really the cause.

Rhinophyma is actually an advanced stage of something called rosacea – a chronic inflammation of the skin. It occurs more often in men than in women. The onset of the initial stage of rosacea typically happens between the ages of 30 and 50. Rhinophyma then develops gradually.

Middle-aged men have the highest risk for developing this condition, according to the journal *American Family Physician*. You are at a higher risk for rosacea—and subsequently rhinophyma—if you have light skin, hair, and eyes. A family history of rosacea is also a risk factor for the condition.

Rhinophyma may respond to medication if diagnosed in its early stages. Some medications are successful in treating a variety of symptoms related to rosacea, including:

- oral antibiotics to reduce inflammation and redness
- topical medications to minimize swelling
- oral isotretinoin, which is used for severe acne – it prevents the sebaceous glands from producing oil.

More usually though, I'm afraid surgery is the preferred, most effective treatment for long term success. Sometimes, the tissue is completely excised and the raw area skin-grafted. There's still a possibility of the 'blossom' slowly growing back after the skin has healed though. And yes, drinking heavily will make it worse.

Taking care of your skin isn't about vanity or being 'pretty'. If looking good matters to you, that's fine. Personally, I reckon I could use a panel beater more than a beautician. But that's not the point. It's about your health.

You can put top quality fuel in the car, clean all of the filters regularly, and drive as carefully as possible, but if you don't look after the exterior – keep it under cover out of the elements when possible, wash and polish regularly – the rust gets in and eventually the bodywork starts to fall apart.

> **Simply put**: your skin is one of the most vulnerable organs in your body to having the effects of ageing made worse by other factors.

3.3 The hard stuff – bone, muscle and fat

It's pretty hard to argue that as we get older there are structural changes to the 'hard frames' of our bodies. One of the reasons for that is that both estrogen and testosterone, and a number of other body chemicals, are important for normal tissue growth and maintenance.

As hormone levels decline the **bones** can deteriorate. One sign of that is a condition called osteopenia, which basically means 'low bone mass'. Osteopenia isn't especially dangerous itself, but it's a big step on the road to osteoporosis.

Also known as 'fragile bone disease', osteoporosis is characterized by a "significant" loss of bone mass. In addition to the hormonal decreases – perhaps even more importantly, there's a deficiency in calcium, vitamin D, magnesium and other vitamins and minerals. Many foods contain these bone-building minerals, so a poor diet can be a factor, too.

If it progresses, osteoporosis can lead to loss of height, stooped posture, humpback, and severe pain.

Osteoporosis is best diagnosed by something called Dual Energy X-ray Absorptiometry or DEXA. This scan uses low-energy x-rays that expose patients to a lot less radiation than standard x-rays. It's a painless, non-invasive procedure usually done on the hip, spine, wrist, finger, shin, or heel.

The scan assesses the calcium levels in the bone. The results are compared to those of healthy individuals and are measured as a "score".

It's called a T-score, and it's worked out by comparing the test result to an average score for a healthy 30-year-old of the same sex and race. 'SD' (Standard Deviation) is a measure of the difference between the patient's score and the benchmark "normal" score.

T-score	What the score means
2.5 to -1 SD	Normal bone density
Between -1 and -2.5	Osteopenia (low bone density)
Below -2.5	Osteoporosis

So if you get one of these DEXA tests done and your score is anywhere below -1, expect your doctor to order some changes to your diet and exercise regime. If it's under -2.5 you can expect some medication to try to increase your bone mass.

Remember though, osteoporosis is a *risk factor*, not a disease. Bone density isn't an absolute indicator that you *will* be breaking bones more often in future. Don't rush out and ask for a DEXA test if you don't have a good reason to.

The biggest clue that you might have a problem is if you are already starting to notice a tendency to break more easily. A knock or bump that in years gone by would have just left a bruise now means a sharper pain where you've cracked the bone. Doctors and x-ray people call it 'minimal trauma fracture'. Of course, if your bones weren't great to begin with you might not notice much difference, but if that's the case it might be worth getting your bone density checked as part of an overall check-up anyway.

Simply put: age and diet can affect bone density, meaning your bones break more easily than they used to. You can get a simple test done if you reckon you might have that problem.

Muscles can suffer from a condition that's the equivalent of osteopenia – it's called sarcopenia. It means a steady loss of lean muscle mass. And as is the case with bones, there can be a number of contributing factors.

Sarcopenia is more common in people who don't get much regular exercise. Physically inactive people can lose 3% to 5% of muscle mass after they hit 30, with the rate of decline getting rapidly worse as they get older.

That doesn't mean being active makes you immune. It can be influenced by diet – too little good quality protein, insufficient calories, too much poor quality protein (which leads to producing too much acid) - can all do damage.

Just getting older has a profound effect. Among the hormones that markedly decline with ageing are things with names out of a spy movie - MGF (mechano growth factor) and IGF-1 (insulin-like growth factor 1). These are critical in maintaining muscle and bone mass. If the levels of these hormones are inadequate, no amount of exercise and good diet will maintain lean muscle mass.

Losing muscle mass can have other effects beside the obvious decrease in strength. Muscle tissue is a kind of metabolic storehouse – it retains and produces proteins and other chemicals for survival and recovery. So you may struggle more and be slower to heal after surgery or any physical trauma because you simply haven't got that much of a 'reservoir' to support your immune system and other recovery systems.

You could also be more prone to getting a hernia. That's when a muscle wall separates and whatever was behind it (a bit of an organ, like your stomach, or maybe another muscle) pokes through.

It needn't be a tear – sometimes the muscle fibres part like a stage curtain. They're not always dangerous. They're not always even painful. But they should always be checked out just in case. If you've got a little bulge somewhere that you didn't used to, show your doctor. If it's a big bulge or a really sore one, see your doctor quick.

Simply put: as you get older it's natural that your body loses muscle mass. That can make you slower to heal and more prone to damage. Diet and exercise can help, but won't necessarily fix the problem.

And then there's **fat**. In general terms, ageing males are prone to loss of muscle mass and a gain in fat mass, especially in the form of what's called visceral or central fat. It's called 'central' because it's in the centre of your body. Other names for it are 'middle age spread' or 'the beer gut'. (In women it generally goes to the hips – it's another fundamental difference between us.)

A 2004 study of blokes aged between 24 and 85 years confirmed that testosterone levels are inversely correlated with the measurement around the waist. Not 'obesity', or overall fat, but quite specifically related to the stuff round the middle. The bigger your gut, the lower your testosterone level is likely to be.

It's a vicious cycle. The question has been which is cause and which is effect. The traditional view was that the fat came first, and that low testosterone was simply the result, as that study seemed to confirm.

The chemistry behind that is that fat tissue is extremely active when it comes to affecting hormones, particularly testosterone and estrogen. 'Aromatase' is an enzyme in fat tissue that converts testosterone into estradiol (which is one of the main types of estrogen). So if there's a lot of aromatase activity being produced by an excess of fat, then that decreases testosterone and increases estrogen levels.

The other side of the coin is evidence that testosterone is tied to a lot of chemistry in different parts of the body. For one thing, it plays a vital role in how our bodies balance the production and management of glucose and insulin.

Decrease the testosterone (which, like I said before, happens slowly but surely with age) and, ultimately, the body stores more sugar – and the place where it stores the sugar is in that deep central fat. And so, to store more sugar, the body packs on more fat.

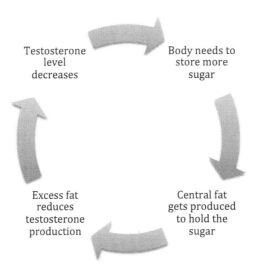

Testosterone level decreases → Body needs to store more sugar → Central fat gets produced to hold the sugar → Excess fat reduces testosterone production →

There's the vicious cycle! Age may be what kick starts it, or there may be something else going on in your body that's either lowering the testosterone or encourageing the fat to build up.

> **Simply put**: ageing doesn't make you fat but it can make the fat harder to shift. And if you're already overweight, that can make the effects of ageing worse.

3.4 Blood lines – take heart

The heart is what keeps us alive, right? Right. The right side pumps blood to the lungs to receive oxygen and get rid of carbon dioxide. The left side pumps oxygen-rich blood to the body. Stop the heart for long, and you die. Everyone knows that.

And everyone knows that heart disease is one of the biggest killers in the Western world, right? Right. Especially amongst older people.

Now read that again please.

Heart *disease*. Not 'getting older', not 'middle age' or 'mid-life'.

Yes, the heart does go through some changes as we age. It's a muscle, and its cells can deteriorate with time. But it gets the most regular, constant exercise of any muscle in the body.

Normally your heart works at a pretty regular steady rate. There are things that make it work harder than usual:

- Certain medications
- Emotional stress
- Extreme physical exertion
- Illness
- Infections
- Injuries

There are also things we do to our heart that can interfere with its working properly. I don't reckon it's a coincidence that lots of studies have shown that this is more common among people in developed countries and only occurs rarely in the developing countries, except among those who have adopted a 'Western' way of life.

Maybe the stress of modern life is a factor. A big chunk of the blame lies in the fact that too many of us eat too much salt, or too many refined carbohydrates. They definitely cause progressive problems. As they build up in the body, the effects become more obvious and we blame them on getting older. That's unfair on the poor old heart, which is doing the best it can!

The valves of the heart, which control the flow of blood in and out, can stiffen up with age. That's caused by the gradual build-up of a substance called lipofuscin. Lipofuscin is made of microscopically fine granules of oxidized fat. It can also contain sugars and metals like mercury, aluminium, iron, copper and zinc. It's nasty stuff, linked to macular degeneration, Alzheimers and Parkinson's Disease as well as heart trouble.

At the very least, it's one of the main reasons why we know from studies in many Western nations that a person's blood pressure rises as he or she grows older.

Even how you look after your teeth affects your heart. Your mouth is one of the very few parts of your body where there's a blood flow to the heart that *doesn't* go through the filtration of the liver. Bad bacteria that build up in the mouth, in bleeding gums for example, get to the heart and inflame the blood vessels. It's no coincidence that the stuff that builds up on your teeth and the stuff that angiograms identify building up on the walls of the heart arteries share the same name – plaque.

Post-mortem studies of people who've died of heart disease have found a high incidence of the bacteria and germs in the damaged heart also being present in the cadavers' gums. This is something that builds up with time, and it's not uncommon for 'middle age' to be about when the body's reaching some threshold levels, beyond which symptoms start to appear.

Suddenly brushing and flossing properly are about more than avoiding bad breath!

Moving to the other end of the body - I've seen some scare-mongering stuff in the papers and on TV about testosterone replacement treatments being bad for the heart. I went looking for evidence, and found the opposite.

There are over forty studies that have examined the relationship of testosterone levels to the presence or development of coronary heart disease, and none have shown a positive correlation. Many of these studies have found the presence of coronary heart disease to be associated with low testosterone levels.

Again – read that last sentence carefully. "Associated with" – not "caused by". There's more going on than just wearing out with age.

Simply put: Your heart is one of the most vulnerable parts of your body as you get older due to the build-up of stuff in your system – particularly in your blood.

3.5 Sex – the nuts and bolts

In this chapter I'll talk about the physical issues that might occur – the machinery, if you like. Next chapter I'll talk about what can happen to the bloke driving the equipment.

Let's face it, there's enough stuff that can go wrong with a blokc's plumbing to fill a book just with that. Okay, I'll write that one next. For now, I'll just focus on the stuff that is, or is accused of being, age-related.

"**Erectile dysfunction**" it's called on the billboards and ads promoting a range of wonder drugs. It's when you can't get it up (or keep it up) or the old fella just doesn't get as hard as he used to.

"John Thomas says goodnight to Lady Jane, a little droopingly, but with a hopeful heart."

- D. H. Lawrence

Author of 'Lady Chatterley's Lover'

Male sexual arousal is a complex process that involves the brain, hormones, emotions, nerves, muscles and blood vessels. Erection trouble can result from a problem with any of these. Likewise, stress and mental health concerns can cause or worsen it, and we get another vicious cycle: some physical condition (quite possibly minor) interferes with your sexual response, you get anxious about maintaining an erection, and the more anxious you get, the more the problem happens.

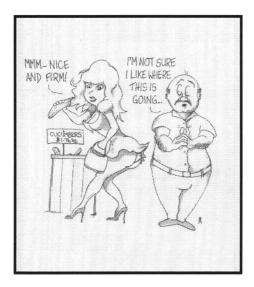

But the root cause (excuse the pun) is most often physical. There are a lot of factors that can cause or contribute to 'erectile dysfunction' on their own, or worse, in combination. Here's a list from the Mayo Clinic:

- Heart disease
- Clogged blood vessels (atherosclerosis)
- High cholesterol
- High blood pressure
- Diabetes
- Obesity
- Metabolic syndrome — a condition involving increased blood pressure, high insulin levels, body fat around the waist and high cholesterol
- Parkinson's disease
- Multiple sclerosis

- Peyronie's disease — development of scar tissue inside the penis
- Certain prescription medications, including antidepressants, antihistamines and medications to treat high blood pressure, pain or prostate conditions
- Tobacco use – over time restricting blood flow to veins and arteries
- Alcoholism and other forms of substance abuse
- Sleep disorders
- Surgeries or injuries that affect the pelvic area or spinal cord
- Certain medical treatments, such as prostate surgery or radiation treatment for cancer
- Injuries, particularly if they damage the nerves or arteries that control erections – sporting injuries are common culprits
- Psychological conditions, such as stress, anxiety or depression
- Prolonged bicycling, which can compress nerves and affect blood flow to the penis, may lead to temporary or permanent erectile dysfunction

Many of those can add to the natural reduction in the hormones maintaining muscle mass that I mentioned earlier, as well as having their own impacts.

"Middle age is when it takes you all night to do once what once you used to do all night."

- Kenny Everett

English disc jockey and comedian.

You might notice that very few of them are "sudden" events. It's the build-up, particularly of things that affect the muscles, nerves and blood vessels, that's the problem. If what you've noticed hasn't been a gradual decline but a sudden change then I reckon you need to be talking to a doctor, and possibly a urologist, ASAP. Seriously.

> **Simply put**: as you get older you're more likely to suffer from one or more of the many things that can make your hard-on less hard.

Some blokes don't have trouble with getting or maintaining an erection, but find they don't come like they used to. Maybe it's too soon, or too little, or not at all – they're all not uncommon **ejaculation problems**.

First up, let's get this clear: ejaculation and orgasm are NOT the same thing. I know it feels like it, but they're really two separate responses to stimulation. One is the body's response, the other one is in your brain.

"Ejaculation" refers to the physical reflex that releases semen, and "orgasm" refers to the *feeling* of climax or pleasure you get as a result of physical and/or psychological stimulation.

For some men (at whatever age after puberty), orgasm and ejaculation both happen, but not at the same time. Some men may ejaculate after orgasm or before orgasm. Some men may not ejaculate at all. Other men might ejaculate but fail to orgasm. None of those things are 'abnormal' or unhealthy – it's just how some blokes' bodies work.

It's when there's a change in that working that there could be a problem. And those changes are more likely to happen, or get noticed, as we hit middle age.

Premature ejaculation – coming too soon – usually with minimal stimulation and certainly before you (and maybe your partner) want it to happen, is something that affects some blokes all their life. For them it starts with pretty much the first time, and then may just keep happening.

But if that's not you: "this didn't used to happen!" you say indignantly (or sadly, or apologetically), then there must be a reason. Something is affecting the sensitivity of the penis or the operation of the plumbing.

'Acquired premature ejaculation' as it's called can arise due to:
Medical conditions such as
- diabetes,
- erectile dysfunction,
- chronic prostatitis,
- an overactive thyroid.
Psychological issues, such as
- relationship problems,
- anxiety,
- stress,
- infrequent sexual activity (or significantly less frequent than it used to be)
- loss of sexual interest by and/or in the partner.

Again, many of these things build up over time rather than being 'sudden onset', although you might only notice the effect suddenly one night!

It's important you realise – *you're not alone*! We don't talk about it much, but researchers who <u>have</u> managed to extract straight answers reckon 20% to 30% of men of all ages suffer from premature ejaculation at some time in their lives.

Alternatively, if the problem is that you feel like you're coming, but nothing comes out, ("dry coming" it's sometimes called) there are two possible conditions responsible.

One is *retrograde ejaculation*, which is when the semen in effect goes backward. This occurs when the bladder neck fails to close at the moment of climax and instead of making its way out, semen passes through the bladder neck into the bladder rather than out where you expect it.

This is an uncommon condition, but it's also physically harmless (although psychologically it can be a worry!).

There are some drugs that can sometimes help, and if there's something really severely wrong, a bit of surgery on the bladder neck might be required. But for the most part, doctors aren't inclined to treat the 'problem' because a.) it's difficult to treat and b.) it's in no way dangerous.

The other condition is called *anejaculation*, which means you don't come at all. That can happen with or without the feeling of having an orgasm.

It's hard to distinguish from retrograde ejaculation – in fact the only way is for a urine sample to be taken soon after sexual climax. The doctor then checks for sperm in the urine. If sperm is found the diagnosis is retrograde ejaculation and if sperm is not found the diagnosis is anejaculation.

There are lots of potential causes for the condition, such as:

- Surgery to the prostate, bladder or abdomen
- Prostatitis, which is the inflammation of the prostate gland
- Conditions affecting the nervous system, such as Parkinson's disease
- Diabetes
- Spinal cord injuries
- Partial blocking to the urethra
- Some drugs can interfere with the ability to ejaculate or orgasm
- Psychological factors such as stress or deep-seated anxieties about sex or the relationship.

The prostate gland enlarges with age as some of the prostate tissue is replaced with a scarlike tissue. This condition, called benign prostatic hypertrophy (BPH) – it's NOT prostate cancer, affects about 50% of men. This may cause problems with slowed urination, as well as with blocking ejaculation.

Your best starting point is to consult your doctor for a physical check to exclude physical causes.

Anejaculation due to partial blockage of the urethra can be treated with surgery, but this is uncommon. Infections that might cause prostatitis can be treated with the right drugs. A lot of doctors though may take the view that if fertility is not an issue (i.e. you've got no pressing urge to have kids) then no medical treatment may be needed.

I reckon if it bothers you, then it's an issue. If you want it fixed, then you've got the right to ask for that to happen. If the physical causes have been ruled out and there's still nothing happening for you, then ask for a referral to a good counselor so you can talk through your concerns and try to find an answer.

For most blokes in their 'middle years' **fertility** isn't an issue any more. But if you *do* want to start or expand a family, then don't put pressure on yourself. (Conversely, if you don't want more kids, don't take it for granted that it can't happen!)

Fertility varies from man to man anyway, and age isn't a good predictor of male fertility. But there are a few age-related things that could be affecting you if you're afraid you're 'firing blanks':

- The gradual decrease in testosterone production.

- The actual mass of the testes themselves decreases.

- The tubes that carry the sperm may become less elastic (a process called sclerosis).

- The epididymis, seminal vesicles, and prostate gland lose some of their surface cells but continue to produce the fluid that helps carry sperm.

That last one means that the volume of fluid ejaculated might remain the same, it's just that there might be fewer living sperm in it.

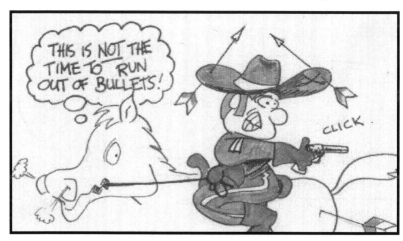

Other than the circumstance I mentioned before of an enlarged prostate blocking ejaculation, prostate function isn't closely related to fertility. A man can father children even if his prostate gland has been removed.

All of these changes usually occur gradually. It doesn't mean fatherhood is beyond you, but if it's your goal and it's not happening then go looking for answers – don't automatically blame your partner, or yourself!

Simply put: Ageing by itself doesn't prevent a man from being able to enjoy sex, but performance can decline over time. If there's a sudden change talk to your doctor, just in case it's a sign of something serious.

3.6 "I'm sick of feeling sick!"

Here's another one of those ugly long words that medical people sometimes throw around – *immunosenescence*.

The technical definition of that is "an age-related decline in lymphoid cell activity".

What *that* means is that as we get older our bodies produce less of the cells and chemicals that fight disease, so we're more likely to pick up any diseases that are going around. Infections, bugs, viruses, whatever – and we're less able to get over them than we used to be.

A winter flu that might lay up a fit twenty-five year old for a couple of weeks could kill his grandfather.

Until recently it was figured that this wasn't really a problem for most people until they were about seventy or older. In the last few years though, the penny has dropped with some doctors and researchers that this 'age threshold' has slipped. People are getting sicker, younger.

The key to the 'killer cells' that fight disease is in the gut. Most of us don't treat our guts as well as we should, or as well as our ancestors did. That's not entirely our fault, as the quality of the food we eat isn't what it used to be. I go into more detail on that elsewhere in this book, but the point is that the good 'killer cells' are declining in production faster and earlier than they used to.

> **Simply put:** 'getting old' doesn't make you sick, but as you age your body is less able to fight off disease.

3.7 Your brain: the odd one out

Memory test: back in Chapter 1, what did I say was exceptional about your brain cells?

Answer: The neurons are the only ones of the five to ten trillion cells in your body that don't die and get replaced every few days or every few weeks. The neurons you grow in childhood are pretty much all you get.

Some extremely clever scientists have apparently succeeded in producing new neurons out of stem cells found in the brain, but I haven't seen any hard evidence that the body actively does that by itself.

There are maybe 100 billion neurons in your brain. They're complex nerve cells, each with a special threadlike fibre called an axon. That's the bit that carries electrical impulses between cells. Some axons are short, just reaching to the next cell along in the brain. Others are much longer and carry impulses down the spinal cord – impulses that do useful things like enable you to walk. Others split and branch into as many as thousands of endings that distribute impulses over lots of cells. Those impulses travel at between nine and four hundred feet per second – the proverbial speed of thought. (The speed of light is a bit over 9.8 feet per second.)

On average, the brain makes up about 2.5% of total body weight. But when you're at rest it's using 22% of the energy that goes on keeping the body ticking over.

I've read that the trillions of connections in the neural network make the human brain "the most complicated object in the universe". Given that there's so much universe we know absolutely nothing about I reckon that's stretching it a bit, but I do like the old observation that if the brain was simple enough to fully understand then we'd be too simple to understand it.

What we do know, though, is that although neurons do die off with ageing, in a healthy brain (i.e. one not affected by something like a stroke or infection) that rate is only gradual. And while the dead cells don't seem to be routinely replaced like they are in the skin or other organs, the living healthy neurons can continue to grow new axons. That means we're capable of learning new things even as we get older.

That's what "rewiring the brain" is all about – you might have read the term. When a stroke victim learns to speak again, they're not growing new brain cells. It's the axons of the surviving healthy cells splitting and branching and linking to other healthy cells, effectively finding their way around the damaged bits.

It's a natural process but not an easy one. It takes effort and encouragement. Sit and stare at a wall all day (or a TV full of stuff that doesn't challenge you to think) and the brain will settle into lines of least resistance.

"First, you forget names. Then you forget to pull your zipper up and finally you forget to pull it down."

- Branch Rickey

US baseball executive & civil rights activist 1881-1965

It's not all plain sailing. Some brain functions do deteriorate, most notably it seems, memory. There are two elements to that. One is a loss of 'storage capacity', the other is the ability to quickly access and use what's in that storage.

There are two types of memory. Long-term memory is the filing cabinet where we keep names, faces, events etc. You draw on them when you need them, sometimes consciously and sometimes automatically e.g. when you're making decisions without being specifically aware that you're drawing on past experiences.

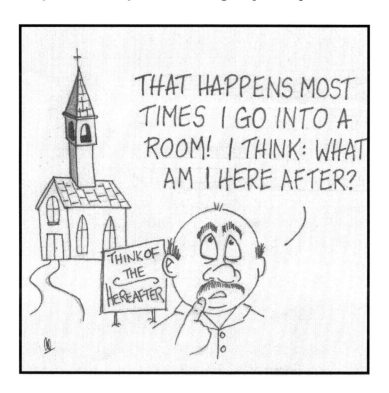

The other type is called 'working' memory. That holds stuff for seconds or minutes while you're *doing* stuff. You remember the last few words or sentences you said, or the last bit of the garden you worked on, or the last ingredients you put in the stew – so that you can complete the conversation or the job at hand. Then the working memory clears, and you go on to the next task.

Either or both type of memory may deteriorate with age. The working memory is probably the more commonly affected, and the most obvious.

It doesn't usually happen in isolation. If your diet isn't adequate or there's a build-up of toxins happening in your body it won't just be your brain that's showing the effects.

"I can remember what happened in High School, but not where I went last Thursday." Sound familiar? Minor problems with memory aren't a big issue, but they can be warning signs that there may be bigger troubles ahead if you don't make an effort to improve your overall health.

Don't blame the poor old brain for failing eyesight or hearing though. It still processes the input perfectly well – it's just that the eyes and ears themselves can lose their edge.

Take the eyes. The way we live now can really damage them. In China about 90% of kids aged 17 to 19 years old are nearsighted. In the 1950's it was more like 10%. Too much time staring at computers, you reckon? Only in part. The real problem is too little time outdoors. Research is showing that exposure to sunlight – not lots of it, but regular – is the best defence against myopia. A 2013 study in Taiwan showed that getting kids outside during their lunch breaks was enough to make a significant difference in preventing eye deterioration. If you spend your day stuck in an office – get out whenever you can!

You can't blame the brain for headaches either. It's one part of the body with no pain receptors. If your head hurts it's coming from the tissues and stuff *around* the brain. It records the pain from everywhere else, but doesn't feel it itself.

Just because it can't register pain doesn't mean it can't be damaged though. Some symptoms are physical, usually showing up in the nervous system or as loss of function in some part of the body. Others though are psychological, and often not recognised as resulting from brain injury or trauma. I'll look at that more closely in Chapter 4.3.

But even though it doesn't register pain, your brain can suffer from inflammation. Bits of it can swell, even microscopically, and be affected by chemicals that ultimately lead to cells deteriorating. That's what underlies things like:

- Autism,
- Epilepsy,
- Multiple sclerosis,
- Parkinson's disease,
- Alzheimer's disease,
- Depression.

You might notice that some of them are conditions that can show up from a very early age but others tend to occur later in life. In those cases it looks a lot like a cumulative effect rather than something that just suddenly 'happens'.

Brain inflammation isn't something that's absent one day and there the next (unless it's the result of injury or infection). If the symptoms are noticed suddenly, it's probably because a threshold has been crossed – the inflammation has reached a point that the brain cells can't deal with any more.

Simply put: your brain is incredibly complex. It's vulnerable to ageing but unless something dramatic happens it's usually a gradual decline.

.o0o.

4 HOW IT MIGHT AFFECT YOUR HEAD

You can't separate the "physical" (menopause/andropause) from the "psychological" (mid-life crisis) because the brain is part of the body. It's a chemical producing organ.

> ## "The chief function of the body is
> ## to carry the brain around."
> *- Thomas Edison*

On average, a bloke's brain accounts for about 2% of his body weight, but about 20% of his blood and oxygen use. Your body knows the brain is important. It runs the show. But what affects one affects the other.

You know it. When you feel crook it's hard to concentrate, you feel flat, or irritable, or unhappy, or all of the above.

On the other side of the coin, you know how your emotions can affect your body. For instance, when you're angry your skin can change colour, your breathing and heart rate change, your fists might bunch up without you consciously noticing.

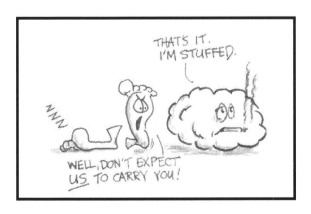

In addition to the physical symptoms I talked about last chapter, the UK National Health Service also list some psychological effects of 'male menopause':

- moodiness/irritability
- reduced concentration span
- loss of enthusiasm
- depression.

Some blokes start to have Regrets for the first time in their lives. For others, what had been little niggles become big concerns. At 36, the world's our oyster. But by 44 we can feel like we're trapped inside the oyster shell, gasping for air.

"You can't help getting older, but you don't have to get old."

- George Burns

American comedian, still doing stand-up at age 100

The stereotype 'Grumpy Old Man' certainly exists – I'm often accused of being him. And there's nothing wrong with that. There's plenty to be grumpy about some days. The problems come when that negative, super-critical attitude takes over your life to the detriment of any good stuff going on.

It becomes self-perpetuating, too. Negative reinforcement. The more you say stuff like "Jeez my life is crap" or "I'm useless at this" or "I'm not the bloke I used to be", the more you train the people around you to believe it. You can't be surprised then when your wife, kids, or boss start telling you the same thing.

"Just try to give your best and try to be better tomorrow than yesterday."

- Arsene Wenger

Manager of Arsenal Football Club, 20+ years

4.1 The roads not taken

Sometimes it's the result of looking at what other blokes have achieved, or the stuff they've got. 'What have they got that I don't? What did *I* do wrong?'

> ## "Comparison is the thief of joy."
> *- Theodore Roosevelt*
> US President 1901 – 1909

Other times the midlife stew often starts with some garden-variety boredom. That's often where the moodiness comes from. If you've been hoeing the same row for twenty years, it's quite reasonable to wonder if there aren't some more interesting rows somewhere else.

That can quickly turn into 'the dangerous wish list'. The Maserati you saw on last night's *Top Gear*. Pipe surfing in Hawaii. The hot blonde working on the third floor.

None of them are necessarily dangerous, although they can be. If you're not The Stig and all you're used to is getting the Mitsubishi round the suburbs then you're a fair chance of wrapping the Maserati round a tree when you misjudge a corner at 130+.

If a four foot swell on the Gold Coast is the limit of your experience, then taking on a North Shore monster could see you putting your head through your surfboard. Or vice versa.

As for the blonde, well, here's a sampler of risks: unpredictable jealous partner (hers or yours), the discovery that your heart isn't as resilient as it used to be, bankruptcy, an interesting venereal disease, crushingly embarrassing public rejection – do I need to go on?

It doesn't mean that ambition is a bad thing. But a man's got to know his limitations. Extend them and push them, sure. That's called growing. One step at a time.

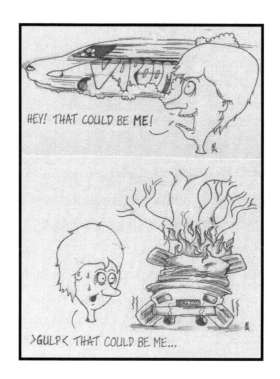

You can't go from jogging around the block one weekend to running a marathon the next.

If you've really *got* to have the sports car, learn to drive it properly, on roads that are built to take the sort of speeds the thing is capable of. If you're going to surf in Hawaii take some advice from the locals. As for the hot blonde... well, the best I can suggest is that you start by taking a good honest look at the mirror, and your bank statement.

Simply put: don't let boredom be the death of you. Trying something new and exciting can be great, but prepare yourself first.

4.2 Staring in the rear view mirror

I remember an old *Peanuts* cartoon. Charlie Brown is visiting Lucy's 'psychiatric advice' stand, worried about his Dad.

"Every night he sits in the kitchen, looking at his old High School Yearbook and sighing," he explains.

Lucy asks how old Dad is, to which Charlie replies, "He's just turned forty, I think."

"Right on cue. Don't worry about it," is her sage five-year-old doctor's advice.

> **"I learned... that one can never go back, that one should not ever try to go back – that the essence of life is going forward. Life is really a One Way Street."**
>
> *- Agatha Christie*
>
> English crime writer

There are a number of elements to this, all related but not quite the same as each other.

There's a remembrance of things lost. The unbeaten ton for the Second XI. The high school sweetheart who ended up marrying a wealthy dentist instead. The big growly motorbike you traded in for the Family Car.

There's the picking over of old mistakes. The marriage you screwed up because you were drinking too much. The critical exam you botched because you didn't really study for it. The times you missed important events in your kid's life because you were too busy working.

And there's pining for opportunities missed, or not noticed at the time. That's not the same as past mistakes, where you pretty much know what the consequences of your actions (or inactions) were. It's a backwards look at those 'roads not taken'. "I should have gone for that overseas job that they offered me." "I shouldn't have ended that relationship." "I should have stayed with the band."

I'm developing an opinion that 'should' is one of the most destructive words in the English language.

"The older we get, the better we used to be."

- John McEnroe

US tennis player and commentator

It's the past. That stuff which has passed. Unless you've got a working time machine, you can't go back and fix, or undo, any of it.

You might be able to address some consequences. If there's someone you owe an apology to, you can make it, if not in person then in some way that works for you. Write a letter and post it in an unaddressed envelope. Have the conversation with a sympathetic mate who'll be the 'surrogate' for whoever you're saying sorry to.

Regrets are like experience – they're only valuable if you learn from them. I've heard it reckoned that history teaches us that we learn nothing from history. I say – buck the trend.

"Any man can make mistakes, but only an idiot persists in his error."

- Cicero

Roman philosopher and statesman, @44 B.C.

A middle-aged man may suddenly decide that much of what he once thought was important now seems trivial and ridiculous. A positive spin on this insight would be to set about discovering what *is* important to him. But too many of us get hung up on the negative without looking for ways to move on.

The most dangerous thing about staring into the rear view mirror is that you lose sight of the road ahead and the conditions around you. If you spend all your time looking back at the past, analysing and re-analysing, losing yourself in memories and 'what-if' games, then you'll never be able to apply any lessons you might learn.

Instead, you risk making a bunch of new mistakes and building a new catalogue of regrets by failing to appreciate the things you've got now and doing nothing positive about your future.

> **Simply put**: the biggest danger of spending too much time regretting the past is that you'll wind up regretting the things you've missed in the present.

4.3 Depression - the black dog that follows you around

Depression isn't exclusively a "middle age" thing. One look at the youth suicide figures should be enough to tell you that (over 250 Aussie blokes under 25 in 2013, and that's doesn't include overdoses and car crashes). But the years after 40 can often be when it rears its ugly head for the first time.

As if tedium and a sense of loss weren't enough, middle age is often when the first bolts of serious bad news strike. It could be the death of a parent, trouble in a marriage, or a career setback.

If you're a father, it can be the transformation of the 8-year-old who thought you were God into the teenager who thinks you're the devil.

Or it could come from some of the major physical things that may make themselves known. Sudden chest pain or the words "we want to do a biopsy" can get a bloke thinking about what he's done with his life – what he's missed and might be about to miss.

When pro golfer Paul Azinger was told he had bone cancer, this was his reaction:

"It was the first time in my life that I really understood that I wasn't bulletproof. When... you feel like you're at the peak of your career and you've got a great family and more money than you ever dreamed of making, you don't think about dying. I still think of myself as a kid, just a big kid. Now someone was telling me I might die. There's no clever answer when someone tells you that."

It's the accumulation of those negative events and feelings that can push you over the edge of unhappiness into depression.

Not just 'feeling a bit down', but an oppressive feeling that nothing is worthwhile. A feeling that doesn't go away after a good night's sleep, or a few drinks with the mates to cheer us up. A feeling that goes way down deep inside and hangs on, colouring everything else that's going on in our lives. I've heard it described as "anger without the energy".

It's one of the things that us blokes are worst at talking about, yet it's also one of the most common (and dangerous) problems we face.

That's a big part of the trouble – when you're inside it depression feels like the loneliest place on Earth, yet it's really a crowded room. It's just that the people in it don't talk to each other – or anyone else – very much.

I know how it feels. First hand. You recognise (sometimes, or eventually) that there are people who want to help. Especially friends and family. But when you're wrapped in that big black shroud you just don't want anyone getting that close to you – so you wallow.

It's self-indulgent, and self-perpetuating, but that's how it is. I'm not going to lie and say there's an easy way out. If there was, a lot less people would suffer from depression, for a lot less time. A lot less would die.

But it truly isn't hopeless. What a lot of people - especially people who are suffering the effects of depression (either their own, or that of someone they love) – don't realise is that it's a physical condition, not just a psychological one. There's something complex going on inside the brain that makes us feel the way we do.

"Depression is like a bruise that never goes away. A bruise in your mind."

- Jeffrey Eugenides

U.S. novelist, Pulitzer Prize winner

Depression isn't just an imbalance between certain chemicals in the brain, although that's a well researched and recognised part of the problem. Recurrent depressions seems to be more like a degenerative disease in which some nerve cells and neural connections in the brain are damaged or destroyed. Ultimately, what is affected is your ability to adapt to new situations.

Taken in large doses, antidepressants actually work in ways that otherwise would look like brain damage. The drugs not only alter the equilibrium of certain neurotransmitter chemicals (re-establishing the right balance) but also seem to produce changes in the actual structure of numerous neural networks. In other words, they rewire the brain.

Recently there's been research that indicates that some of that physical damage either is, or produces inflammation in the brain. Inflammation is our immune system's natural response to injuries, infections, or foreign compounds.

As a part of that response the body pumps various cells and proteins to the injured or infected site through the blood stream, including a class of proteins called 'cytokines' that facilitate intercellular communication. The new research is finding that people suffering from depression are loaded with these cytokines.

The few clinical trials done so far have found that adding anti-inflammatory medicines to antidepressants not only improves symptoms, it also increases the proportion of people who respond to treatment, although more trials will be needed to confirm this. There is also some evidence that omega 3 and curcumin, an extract of the spice turmeric, might have similar effects. Both are available over the counter and might be worth a try, although as an add-on to any prescribed treatment – there's definitely not enough evidence to use them as a replacement.

The fact that 'normal,' healthy people can become temporarily anxious or depressed after receiving an inflammatory vaccine — like a typhoid shot — lends further credence to the theory.

When you consider that the longer we live, the more we're exposed to a range of things that can knock the brain-box around, it makes sense that depression as a symptom of inflammation becomes more common in older blokes. Look at the issues that bedevil so many ex-boxers, wrestlers and footballers for example.

Former Queensland rep rugby league player Chris Walker is one who's suffered from both depression and anxiety attacks. He reckons,

> "The problem with guys is that they don't want to talk about their problems, then all of a sudden it's too late. They don't want to look vulnerable. They bottle it up and then one day it can spill over and become too much."

Yet as we've just seen it's not about being vulnerable or weak, it's about being damaged. It's because we've all got our own individual body chemistry that some blokes can seem more durable than others. Some blokes cop one knock, or maybe suffer one brief illness and it triggers a self-perpetuating condition that plagues them for the rest of their life.

Others spend years taking large or small bumps to the head without showing obvious effects. I remember years back meeting a pro wrestler named Chris Benoit. "The Canadian Crippler" as he was known was one of the best in the business ever. Not a huge guy, he didn't fit the 'larger than life' mould of the Eighties and Nineties. He was a world champion who got there on sheer bloody toughness, ability, and training hard to be the best he could be.

One of his signature moves was a flying headbutt off the top rope onto his laid-out opponent. Looked spectacular, but it meant several times per week he was knocking his brain around. Even if he didn't hit his forehead on the mat (or his opponent) his skull was being rattled by the dive and impact of landing.

When I met Chris he made it very clear that the only thing that mattered more to him in life than his profession was his family. As much as he loved wrestling ("It's all I really know how to do well," he admitted) he was even more devoted to his wife and son.

Then one awful day he killed them, and himself. Nobody really knows why. There's a thought that maybe his wife had threatened to leave him and take their son with her. Drugs got blamed, not completely unfairly, but I reckon it's more significant that his autopsy showed Chris had sustained so many head traumas over the years his brain showed all the physical signs of major clinical depression.

"So you try to think of someone else you're mad at, and the unavoidable answer pops into your little warped brain: everyone."

- Ellen Hopkins

U.S. novelist

Go back to Chris Walker's comment. "They bottle it up and then one day it can spill over and become too much." If Benoit's condition had been recognised (especially by the man himself) and treated, he and his family might still be alive today.

One in eight men in Australia have been diagnosed with depression. I'd be willing to bet that the figure would be even higher if more blokes were honest with themselves and their doctors. Like I said – it feels lonely but it's a very crowded room.

Drugs and therapies may not address the trigger of your depression – the loss of a loved one or a job for instance – but they can help manage the physical and chemical aspects so it's less likely to spiral out of control.

Simply put: there are things about depression that can be treated, which might break the destructive cycle. But that can only happen when you admit the problem and look for help.

You have to show some support and appreciation for yourself. If you don't nobody else will. A lot of blokes don't like to 'big-note' themselves (although there are plenty who are more than keen to do so). That's okay.

But there's a big difference between being humble and being self-destructive. Self-analysis and self-criticism are fine, but keep the criticism constructive. Otherwise, you become your own trigger for depression.

4.4 Stress responses – the five F options

Stress can be a trigger for depression, but they're not the same thing. Depression is something wrong, both psychologically and, as we've seen, physically. Stress is normal – it's how we handle it that can be a problem.

It goes right back to the days when our ancestors had to spend a lot of their time either hunting for food to eat, or avoiding being eaten by either fighting or running away. They were our main sources of stress for a very long time, and our bodies have deeply ingrained reactions. The reactions known best are 'fight or flight' but there are three others that we also sometimes resort to.

FIGHT: charge at the tiger, shouting and waving your spear;

FLIGHT: run away and try to be faster than the tiger;

FREEZE: stay still, hope the tiger doesn't see you and that it goes away;

FIDGET: look at anything but the tiger, pretend it's not there and maybe it won't be;

FAWN: go pat the tiger and try to make friends with it.

This is the classic example of how what goes on in your head directly affects the body. The stress response is made up of two major parts – two systems that kick in when something happens that makes your head yell, "Stress!!"

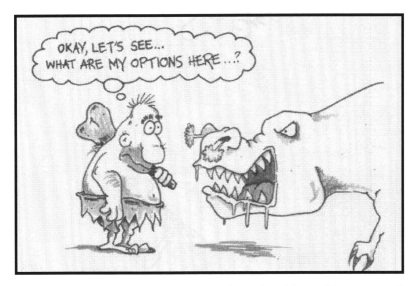

I'll go into detail in a minute but here's a checklist of how your body reacts to stress:

- Heart rate increases

- Pupils dilate

- Body sweats, particularly the hands

- Metabolism increases

- Immune system shuts down

- Digestion shuts down

- Reflexes improve

- Reaction time decreases

On the one hand, you have the autonomic nervous system (ANS), which conscripts two hormones, epinephrine and norepinephrine (also known as adrenaline and noradrenaline), to do the bulk of the work. These two chemicals are released from the adrenal glands and run around the body, making your heart race, opening up your pupils and making your palms all sweaty. In other words, getting your body ready to fight or run away.

They also do some more subtle things, like increasing your metabolism (you'll need that energy whether you're fighting or fleeing) and starting to suppress the immune system (why worry about catching a cold when there's, let's say, a giant bear in front of you). The ANS is responsible for acute and immediate stress response.

The other half of the stress response is the even more messily-named hypothalamic-pituitary-adrenal (HPA) axis. The HPA axis is a very clever self-regulatory network, the main product of which is cortisol.

Cortisol is another hormone, and it also comes from the same part of the brain as epinephrine and norepinephrine. Like them, it increases metabolism and diverts energy from lower-priority body functions like digestion and the immune system. It's of more pressing importance to avoid becoming food than to digest last night's meal.

Combines with adrenaline it actually improves your reflexes and enables you to react faster, which makes sense in a 'fight or flight' situation.

However, its effects last longer than the other two hormones. It hangs around in the body to sustain whichever decision has been made – fighting or fleeing.

Thereby hangs the problem. Back when we wore skins and fought with big sticks, once the decision had been made the resolution was fairly quick. You got away, or won, or you didn't. If you survived, your brain sent a message to suppress the HPA axis so your body could get back to operating normally.

Now though, many of the things that trigger our stress responses don't resolve themselves so readily. A close call with a speeding car while you're crossing the street might leave you taking a deep breath

and getting on with your day, but the stress of preparing to address a board meeting, arguing with the wife, or trying to convince your boss you deserve a pay rise persists a lot longer. You spend hours turning the event over in your head – mentally freezing and staring at it.

Even the things we do to 'relax' and distract ourselves can generate stress reactions in the body – reading gruesome horror stories, watching crime or action movies or TV shows full of suspense, playing blood'n'guts video games, the tense excitement of watching sports, even our reactions to the nightly news (which rarely if ever seems to feature anything *good* to tell us!) – nothing truly restful in there.

That's like 'fidgeting' with stress. Looking the other way, pretending that the problem's not there, but winding yourself up over *something* anyway.

That leads to what we now call 'chronic stress' and that can cause all sorts of problems. Just a few for example:

- Muscle wastage
- Hypoglycemia, when the sugar in the blood isn't processed properly
- Poor digestion, leading to ulcers or colitis
- Compromised immune system

The 'improvement' in reflexes actually becomes a bad thing when it doesn't switch off. Actions and reactions happen without thinking.

"Sorry, honey. Sorry kids. I didn't mean to snap." But you're 'snapping' more often, and snapping harder. It's one of the things stress does.

"If *A* is a success in life, then *A* equals *x* plus *y* plus *z*. Work is *x*; *y* is play; and *z* is keeping your mouth shut."

- Albert Einstein

Physicist, originator of the Theory of Relativity

The 'fawning' response to stress may seem like a strange concept to many, but there are people who embrace their anxieties. They're like adrenalin junkies – "being on the edge lets me know I'm alive" is the sort of comment you might hear. (Personally, breathing does that for me.) Time spent unwinding, or not working, is regarded as wasted time.

I'm prepared to believe that there are people with that approach to life who enjoy long and healthy lives. But they're not in the majority, I reckon. A much greater proportion are the ones who suddenly hit a wall marked 'heart attack', 'burst ulcer' or 'stroke'.

It's probably no coincidence that 'chronic stress' is very much identified with 'Western society'. As countries like India and China and Brazil have increasingly embraced the same sort of high pressure, industrialised and market driven society, the people there are more commonly being diagnosed with 'stress related' illnesses.

The main issues with stress as we get older are that:

- We feel like we have to deal with it more often
- We don't deal with it as easily as we used to
- Both of the above!

All of that is true for a lot of blokes. The lifestyles we lead do create situations that stress us. Getting older can bring more responsibilities – like a growing family, and a job where you're expected to be a supervisor and not just a talented or hard worker.

And the effects accumulate. The cortisol builds up, and while the body does eventually get rid of it, damage is done in the meantime and can often be made worse before it's had time to repair.

To overcome stress and protect your health you've got to make that time. Switch off. Convince your body that the threat has passed by doing something completely different – *fun*, even! It's failing to do that (and lots of blokes reckon they're too busy to allow themselves that break) which moves stress into something unhealthy.

Simply put: stress and its effects on the body are normal. We have a problem when we don't allow ourselves time to recover from stress so the body can't heal.

4.5 Sleep – who needs it?

Some movers and shakers have long bragged of their ability to only sleep four to five hours a night or less and still achieve 'great things'. Donald Trump springs to mind.

For a small number of people, this might even be true. I keep saying it: we all have our own unique body chemistry.

For the great majority of us though, a period of six to eight hours of sleep is *required* every twenty-four hours, even if we don't actually feel 'sleepy'.

There's plenty of research that shows a rested and resilient brain performs better, is better able to regulate emotions and think creatively. If you're normally a good sleeper you probably also know how crappy you feel after a bad night, and worse if you get a couple of them in a row.

The fundamental reason why is that sleep actually cleans the brain.

All of the cells in our body require nutrients and produce waste. Blood vessels supply these nutrients throughout the body, and lymphatic vessels collect the waste from all parts of the body except one - the brain.

That "brain waste" is cleared by the cerebrospinal fluid, which is the quite thick liquid that sits around your brain and spinal cord, and filters *through* the brain while you're asleep.

Previously, scientists thought the brain only cleaned itself by trickling toxins through brain tissues, but researchers now believe wastes are forcefully pushed through the brain at a much faster and higher pace, doing the job more effectively in the tight space inside the skull. A 2013 study even found "hidden caves" open up in the brain while we sleep, allowing this cerebrospinal fluid to flush neurotoxins through and into the spinal column in copious amounts.

The whole process takes six to eight hours to be done properly. Maybe Donald Trump's system works quicker than most people's for some reason. Lucky Donald. Or maybe there's actually something wrong with his brain. Let's not go there.

So while, in general the cerebrospinal fluid acts like the lymphatic system what is important is that this waste clearance only happens while sleeping.

This is the most compelling answer to the question why sleep is so important to the normal functioning of the brain.

The waste products that are filtered through the brain prevent neurological illnesses like Alzheimer's and Parkinson's. One of the most significant of these toxins is a protein called beta-amyloid. It's been found in clumps in the brains of people with Alzheimer's disease. Not surprisingly then, research is indicating that this particular toxin seems to be directly linked with memory loss.

As it turns out, beta-amyloid also works to prevent your body from getting the rest it needs, creating something of a vicious cycle for the chronically sleep-deprived. The more beta-amyloid you have in certain parts of your brain, the less deep sleep you get. And the less deep sleep you have, the less effective you are at clearing out this bad protein, so the more it builds up.

Here's another piece of research that might disturb some of you. Sleeping next to your smartphone - the one that emits 3G and 4G signals all night - affects your brain patterns. It appears that the radiation is actually restructuring your brain cells to the point that it's interfering with the cerebrospinal fluid cleaning out waste material properly.

Research published in 2007 found that the electrical radiation emitted from 'smart' devices is picked up by electrodes inside our brains. Scientists are still trying to figure out just what damage (and exactly how much) the electromagnetic signals emitted from WiFi equipment can actually do to the human brain. But it does look like that just by being in close proximity they're potentially preventing our brains from flushing beta-amyloid.

Simply put: we need good regular sleep to keep our brains working. Lack of sleep means building up chemicals that cause memory loss and more serious conditions.

4.6 Sex – mind over matter

Libido. Sex drive. Not the ability to have sex, but the *desire* to. It changes over time for most people, male and female. And because every person is different it often doesn't change at the same rate for two partners, which can make the problem worse.

To complicate it further, the change doesn't go in the same direction for everyone – not for a while at least.

I'm not talking about physical issues. That was last chapter. This is about what's going on in your mind.

Most commonly, the problem is when all the bits work but you've **lost interest** in doing anything with them.

Let's face it – the brain is our biggest sex organ. Despite accusations that some blokes think with their crotch, the truth is that sexual excitement starts in the brain. That's why and how pornography works – the eyes, the ears, the imagination, the memory even, work together to stimulate below the belt.

There are a lot of things that can get in the way of that, especially as we get older:

- Depression;
- Anxiety;
- Stress;
- Loss of interest from/in a partner (you know what they say about familiarity);
- Demands of work and family.

"I'm too tired" and "I'm too busy" are passion killers, whether it's you or your partner groaning those phrases more often than you want.

It may just be a breakdown in communication between the two of you. One wants more than the other does, which means one person feels pressured (threatened, even) and the other is frustrated and unsatisfied. It's called 'Mis-matched Libidos' or 'Sexual Drive Incompatibility' and it's a recognised disorder in couples that requires its own treatment and therapy options.

Most of these involve counseling of some sort to address the situation where partner A places demands on partner B that B thinks are excessive. So B feels smothered by A and is increasingly unable to meet what they consider demands for sex.

In turn, A feels rejected and unappreciated when what they think have been reasonable, if optimistic requests are repeatedly turned down. It can lead to them either 'looking elsewhere' or losing their self-esteem and losing their own interest in sex.

"The total amount of undesired sex is probably greater in marriage than in prostitution."

- Bertrand Russell

British philosopher and writer, 1872 - 1970

There's a condition called "*Hypoactive Sexual Desire Disorder*" (HSDD). This is defined in textbooks as "the absence of sexual fantasies, thoughts, and/or desire for, or receptivity to, sexual activity, which causes personal/interpersonal distress". Translated: the person has lost interest in sex and isn't happy about it.

A therapist or counselor will look for three criteria to diagnose HSDD:
- Lack of sexual fantasy and desire to engage in sexual activity
- This absence of fantasy and desire must produce marked personal or interpersonal distress. The distress can affect both partners.
- That the disorder isn't actually a result of a major psychiatric or medical condition, or of substance abuse.

If all those boxes get ticked, especially that last one (i.e. there's no physical disorder causing the apparent lack of interest) then the usual next step is therapy and/or counseling. That can be for the individual or the couple if there's a partner involved.

Sex therapy or counselling may include some of the following:

- Cognitive Behavioural Therapy (CBT)
- Anxiety reduction/desensitization
- Psychoeducation
- Enhancing communication
- Addressing fears, conflict and anger
- Behavioural assignments/homework exercises

None of those are scary, freaky or weird, okay? They might be surprising, or challenging, but they might turn out to be fun, too.

If you've got this problem, get this – you're not alone. HSDD is a common problem brought to family counselors, psychologists and sex therapists. It's estimated that about 20% of men are affected by low or absent sexual desire. While sexual interest problems tend to be much less prevalent in men than in women, they do seem to increase with age.

I've read that the man with low sexual interest is often far less troubled by the condition than is his partner. I grant that a woman may not only feel the lack of physical affection and touch, but be worried about the prospects of starting or expanding a family (especially when either or both partner is still fairly young). That's not an exclusively feminine concern though. It's just that it's something (else) we blokes don't talk about much.

Maybe if we did, then the people who write the guidebooks and texts for the therapists would take it more seriously. If not enough of us tell them there's a problem, how can we expect them to look for answers?

Less common but potentially just as much of a problem is the other extreme – when you **just can't get enough** sex.

For some guys it seems to be an urge to over-compensate 'before it's too late'. A way of saying, "I'm not getting old – look!"

The idea of being 'addicted to sex' is a controversial one. At one end of the argument are those who reckon that diagnosis "makes problems of nonproblematic experiences, and as a result pathologizes people" – in other words, it's psychologists creating work for themselves.

At the other end are the likes of the American Society of Addiction Medicine (ASAM), the largest medical consensus of physicians dedicated to treating and preventing addiction. In 2011, ASAM redefined addiction as a chronic brain disorder. That for the first time broadened the definition of addiction from just substances to include addictive 'reward-seeking' behaviors, such as gambling, video gaming and sex.

Their findings are that there's something 'different' going on in the brain. Their research shows that the disease of addiction affects neurotransmission and interactions within reward circuitry of the brain. That leads to addictive behaviors dominating over healthy behaviors.

As a part of that, memories of previous experiences with food, sex, alcohol, drugs or whatever trigger the craving and the renewal of addictive behaviors. Meanwhile, brain circuitry that governs impulse control and judgment is also altered in this disease, resulting in the dysfunctional pursuit of rewards without due consideration to any other consequences.

All of which is fine (if you're okay with self-destructive behavior) until someone else is affected by the addiction. When the addict is so out of control they don't care who they hurt.

The chairman of ASAM said,

> "Simply put, addiction is not a choice. Addictive behaviors are a manifestation of the disease, not a cause. (However) Choice still plays an important role in getting help. While the neurobiology of choice may not be fully understood, a person with addiction must make choices for a healthier life in order to enter treatment and recovery. Because there is no pill which alone can cure addiction, choosing recovery over unhealthy behaviors is necessary."

A lot of chronic diseases require behavioral choices. People with heart disease have to choose whether or not to eat healthier or begin exercising, in addition to undergoing any medical or surgical treatments.

As with problems of low sex drive, much of the available treatment is in the form of counseling and therapy. Calling it an 'addiction' is not a valid excuse for anti-social behavior, far less forcing yourself on anyone. If you're starting to think you've got a problem keeping a lid on your libido talk to someone. Get a referral to a therapist. Explaining yourself to them may not be easy, but it's better than trying to explain yourself in court.

Simply put: the desire for sex changes in everyone over time. That's normal. If it's bothering you or causing problems in your life (or someone else's) the best thing to do is talk to a counselor or therapist.

.o0o.

5 GETTING IN EARLY – LIVE BETTER FOR LONGER

Before I start exploring what options are out there for blokes who are hitting middle age and starting to really notice various symptoms, I want to have a look at what you might be able to do if you haven't yet got that many miles on the clock.

> **"To cure disease after it has appeared is like digging a well only when one feels thirsty, or forging weapons only after the war has begun."**
>
> *- Huangdi Neijing*
>
> 2nd Century B.C. Chinese medical textbook

As far as I can make out, the only way to avoid getting older is to die.

But getting older isn't the same as "getting *old*". I make that point especially if you're one of those blokes who's got it fixed in his head that old equals broken down, worn out and falling apart. It doesn't have to mean that.

Remember what I said earlier about the imaginary car you got when you turned seventeen – the car you could never replace. The better it's maintained, the more care you take with what gets put into it, the better it'll run and the longer it'll last.

5.1 You are what you eat: Food

Here's a curious thing. The incidence of menopause – female or male – is way lower in Japan than most other parts of the world. Apparently that's because the average Japanese person consumes a LOT of soy from an early age. That has the effect of lowering their estrogen level right across their entire life, to a point below what's usual in the 'West'.

So the 'crash' that comes with ageing is from a lesser height and thus much less noticeable.

I'm not suggesting that you start slopping buckets of soy sauce over everything you eat. It probably wouldn't work. Japan is different because the soy consumption starts very young and continues over the whole lifetime.

Clearly though, the things we eat profoundly influence the way our bodies work, especially when those eating 'habits' start young and then continue on through adulthood.

Equally clearly, just because we're all the same species that doesn't mean we all require exactly the same foods in exactly the same proportions.

There are obvious differences like food intolerances and allergies. A good mate of mine has a medical condition that means he has to eat lots of cooked tomatoes to make up for a particular chemical his body doesn't produce enough of. If I eat a pizza that's had too much tomato paste put on it, my knees blow up like footballs – gout.

Your own individual body chemistry means you'll process things a bit differently to me, and to the bloke next to you in the pub, and the bloke across the road, and your cousin living in another country. So all of us need different stuff coming into our systems. Not radically different, but not 100% identical either.

That said, there are some basic essentials that we all need. It's just that the precise quantities vary from person to person, and the best food items to deliver those essentials can also vary.

There's an old saying: "You are what you eat." It's more complicated than that. We are what we digest, assimilate and absorb. A fair percentage of what we eat goes in one end and out the other.

If everything worked perfectly – both diet and digestion – our bodies would get absolutely everything we need from our food. All good stuff, no bad, and no need for anything more. If it ever worked that way it certainly doesn't now.

That's a product of the quality of the food we now eat – individual bad choices, and some poor quality stuff even when we try to choose well.

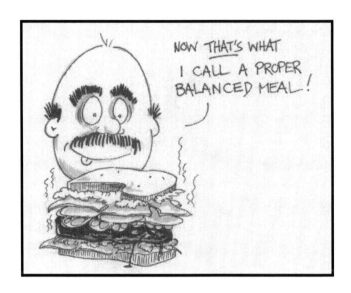

It doesn't help that there's an ENORMOUS amount of stuff being written about what we should and shouldn't be eating, and that a lot of it seems contradictory.

For example, I've got two texts sitting open in front of me right now. One says to avoid the animal fats in meat and milk products because they're full of bad cholesterol that narrows the blood vessels, promoting heart attack and stroke – vegetable fats are the fountain of youth for the circulatory system, it says.

The other book tells me that the most important things we can eat are animal and fish proteins, which our bodies are designed to extract, digest and use most easily.

Helpful, eh? They're both right in their way, but you've got to really look at the detail, and then find the right balance.

So let's take it right back to basics.

Protein is the single most essential part of our diet. When someone dies of 'starvation', what actually kills them is the lack of protein. To keep itself going the body first drains all the energy it can from the fat reserves, however little or much there may be. When that's gone, the muscle tissue gets sapped of energy – critically, including the heart muscle.

How it works is that proteins get broken down into amino acids, and those create some very important components of your body:

- Muscles,
- Immune system cells,
- Neurotransmitters in the brain.

Compromise any of them for any length of time and you won't last long.

Sugar and starch are **carbohydrates**. Sugars are things like glucose, fructose, sucrose, lactose and maltose that have a relatively simple molecular structure. Starches are more complex, made up of long chains of simple sugars.

All carbohydrates ultimately get broken down into glucose during digestion – what varies is how long that takes. Starch breaks down quickly, effectively dumping a load of sugar into your blood in one hit.

Too much sugar in the blood can actually damage the blood vessels, so your pancreas (assuming it's working properly) is quick to produce insulin that picks up the sugar and transports it to the liver and muscles where it's converted into glycogen. From there, it's the raw material for energy and gets burned off.

That's why we need some carbs in our diet – and the more active you are (be it exercise or work) the more essential it is to have the right amount of sugar to burn.

The trouble is, your muscles and liver can only hold so much glycogen. When they're full, the glucose gets dumped into the fat cells. These have a terrific capacity to expand, and are much slower to release the stored sugar than the muscles!

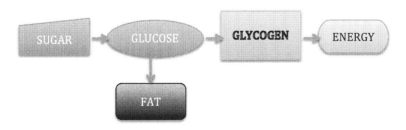

We hear a lot about **cholesterol**, much of it pretty dire. But cholesterol is important to us. For one thing, your body uses different enzymes to convert cholesterol in your bloodstream into various hormones. Your testosterone is made from cholesterol.

Twenty-five percent of the body's cholesterol is stored in the brain, where it's needed to keep that vital organ working properly.

We get it from two sources. The body makes it – your liver should theoretically make most if not all the cholesterol you need. And it comes from food (specifically, food that's sourced from animals) that 'tops up' any shortfall in production.

The problem comes when you get too much cholesterol accumulating in your blood. It's like an overload. The amount released actually decreases, so for example less testosterone gets made.

"I carry a concealed weapon - high cholesterol. It's deadly!"

- Jarod Kintz

US writer

That accumulation happens naturally over time, but too many of us accelerate it by what we eat and how we exercise (or don't).

Cholesterol doesn't dissolve in the blood. It gets 'transported' by carriers called lipoproteins (which are a combination of fat and protein). These come in two types: 'good' and 'bad'.

The 'bad' stuff is low density lipoprotein (LDL). What's bad about it is that it tends to stick to the walls of ateries and clog them, leading to heart attack, stroke and blood clots. Nasty.

The 'good' version is high density lipoprotein (HDL) which carries the cholesterol where it's supposed to go, and also carries LDL away from the arteries and back to the liver to be flushed out of the body. That's when all the quantities are in balance, anyway. Too much LDL is another system overload that isn't good for the quality or length of your life.

LDLs are most often found in foods that are heavy in either 'saturated' fats (poultry skin, fatty red meat, egg yolk, full fat dairy) or 'trans' fat. You'll see this on a label as "partially hydrogenated oil" – it's man made fat that turns up in a lot of processed foods, notably margarine and 'fast' foods.

The good HDL is in unsaturated fat – avocados, seeds, almonds, walnuts, fish, and pure oils like olive, coconut and flaxseed.

Another thing the body needs that gets some bad press is **salt**.

Let's be crystal clear (sorry) – it is an essential. Table salt is made up of about 40% sodium and 60% chlorine. Sodium helps control your fluid balance. That means the fluid inside the cells and outside the cells. It affects blood pressure. It influences the body's function to either hold onto extra fluid when you need it or excrete fluid when you don't. Our bodies automatically regulate how much salt, or sodium, there is present. If levels are too high we get thirsty and drink - this speeds up the elimination of salt through our kidneys.

By being so involved in how fluid moves in and out of cells, sodium also effectively helps to control the way your muscles and nerves work.

So it's not a bad thing. Until there's too much of it, then you run a serious risk of high blood pressure, osteoporosis, kidney trouble and heart disease.

You do lose salt through sweat – on average though, it's about 180 milligrams (mg) of sodium per day unless you perspire really heavily. That's not a lot to replace. Between what you sweat out and what your body naturally uses, the average bloke only needs a minimum of 250 to 500 mg daily to stay at the right level.

The US National Academy of Sciences recommends a maximum of 2400 mg of salt (that's 2.4 grams – always read the label carefully!) per person per day. A teaspoon is 2000 milligrams. The average American takes in between 3500 and 7000 mg per day. A lot of that is not what's sprinkled on the meals.

It's added in the cooking, and it's added in the processing. A half-cup serving of store-bought potato salad, for example, contains 625 mg of sodium, which is more sodium than four slices of bacon (548 mg). Careful label reading is the best way to track your sodium intake.

Oh, and by the way, there's pretty much the same amount of sodium in sea salt as there is table salt. The main differences are flavour and texture (table salt is more highly processed), and that sea salt usually has a few extra minerals in it, although not enough to make any real nutritional difference.

> **Simply put:** protein, carbs, cholesterol and salt are all good and important parts of your diet. The key thing is to get enough of all, and not too much of any. Read the labels!

The best sources of protein are **meat**, eggs and fish (including shellfish). What about the fats and LDL that we know to avoid? The answer is to avoid the fat. Look for lean steaks and cuts of meat. Trim your chops and your bacon and take the skin off the chicken. Steer away from deep-frying, because most of the oils and a lot of the batters aren't doing you any favours.

That still leaves plenty of cooking alternatives:

- steaming
- grilling
- broiling
- roasting
- baking
- boiling
- dry pan frying
- sautéing.

There ought to be a few options there that can work for you.

The other important thing is the quality of the meat. The more processing it's had, the less good for you it's likely to be. And yet, the average 'Western' diet is now reckoned to be made up of 75% processed food – with four to five kilos of food additives consumed per person per year!

Those additives are a cocktail of preservatives, colourings and flavour enhancers. Any of them might be harmless, but individually or in combination with some of the others they might equally well be dangerous to at least some people consuming them.

(A big part of the danger is that some of these additives have only been around for a few years. There hasn't been the chance to test their long-term effects.)

Some of the chemicals trigger allergies or 'food sensitivities' in some people. Sulfites cause no reaction at all in some people, but in others they can set off anything from a skin rash to a life-threatening asthma attack.

Others are just plain toxic. Ammonium acetate is sometimes used as a meat preservative, despite the fact that there's evidence showing it causes cancer in humans – it's just the amount of the stuff that's being argued about!

A good basic rule is to buy fresh. The fewer steps between the farm and the butcher's shop the better. If it's mince, sausages or hamburger patties, ask the butcher what he's put in them besides meat (or read the label, if you're in the supermarket).

Having said that, I have to point out that not all of these chemical additives are applied directly to the meat. Some go in 'second hand', like the formaldehyde that's used as a preservative in some animal feeds, and then turns up in your steak! There's no foolproof answer, but labels like 'organic' and 'grass fed' are about the best guides you can look for. 'Halal' is usually a good indicator of well-prepared meat – ignore any religious connotations that aren't relevant to you and please accept that there is <u>no</u> evidence that halal butchers or abattoirs are funding global terrorism.

Meat is good for you. Good meat is better. It's not essential – if you want to go vegetarian that's your choice – but together with fish it's the best and most easily digestible source of the protein that <u>is</u> essential.

If you're going to make **fish** a big part of your diet, try to make cold-water fish like salmon, trout and cod your first pick. They tend to be higher in omega-3 fats.

They're the good ones. They regulate insulin production, which is what ultimately is responsible for turning sugar into energy. Remember?

Your body doesn't produce its own omega-3 acids. It needs them to get them from food.

Fish is also a good source of protein.

All the points I made above about additives in meat hold true for fish, too. Processed fish (fish sticks, fish cakes, fish fingers etc.) have stuff added in, and in some cases stuff taken out. Some of what's removed can sometimes be what you most wanted to keep.

Shellfish are excellent. They're especially low in unhealthy saturated fats and well stocked with omega-3. Some people suffer from allergies of varying intensities – you probably already know if oysters make you sick or prawns make you break out in itchy spots!

Fish are even more vulnerable than grazing animals to picking up toxins. So much crap gets dumped into the rivers and seas, it's no wonder that we get fish loaded with mercury and heavy metals coming up in nets and on lines.

Some sources are worse than others. Fish from Asia have a bad reputation. Tilapia from China especially so – it's been reported that they use the fish to clean their rivers and streams of human faeces, won't allow the fish to be sold domestically, but happily export it to the rest of the world. Most people would, I suspect, be unhappy to learn they were eating the shit of China...

Farmed fish in general has problems – particularly when the farms are big, mechanized and overcrowded. Those conditions mean the fish are more susceptible to disease, so they get loaded with antibiotics, many of which aren't good for human consumption. Likewise the pesticides that get poured in with the fish (for things like sea lice).

If you don't catch your own, try to buy local – as local as possible. If there is anything nasty being found in the fish caught near where you live you're much more likely to hear about it.

There seems to be a good argument that **cereals and grains** become less important as we get older. Great when we're young, but some of the chemicals they contain don't seem to be processed as well by ageing bodies.

Maybe several generations ago, long after they stopped being hunter/ gatherers and became farmers, some of our ancestors lived on a staple diet of maize or corn flour, supplemented by whatever meat and veg they could find. But as far as we can tell most of them didn't live as long as we do on average.

Grains are high in starch. Your body converts starch into glucose very quickly, which causes a blood sugar spike. That's why some breakfast cereals are promoted as giving you a flying start to the day – it's an energy hit. It gets used up just as quickly, so the spike gets followed by a crash.

At worst, that means fatigue, lethargy – in extreme cases, passing out. Especially when the cereal is most if not all of the breakfast. It's why some kids, and adults, lose concentration mid-morning. Coffee might feel like it helps but it really isn't doing your body any long-term favours.

If you really want to include cereals in your diet, try to avoid the "instant" varieties. They're loaded with extra salt. Instant oatmeal can have up to 360mg of some sort of sodium compound per serve. The same serve of 'pure' oats has none.

These days we more commonly eat grain after it's been processed – ground and baked. Whatever goodness there was in the grain is often refined out, and replaced with salt and sugar to make the bread (or whatever) "taste better". For 'better' read: 'more like what we've come to expect in the last few decades'.

We're seeing more and more "gluten free" labeling and yes, there are people who really do have an intolerance of gluten. Coeliac disease does certainly seem to be diagnosed more often than it used to be.

But now the research is starting to show that for many, the uncomfortable symptoms of bloating, excessive farting, stomach cramps and other gastric discomforts are actually reactions to other stuff. Yeast. Sugar. Additives. Possibly there's a reaction to a particular combination of ingredients. And for some, it's a cumulative thing – like their body has a threshold of a substance beyond which they get a bad reaction. That's one reason why some blokes develop these symptoms as they get older.

It takes specialist testing to know exactly what's being reacted to. Not every GP thinks to make that referral. Not every bloke knows to ask for it (even amongst those blokes who will talk to the GP about their intestines). But if you feel like your gut expands by an inch or three every time you have a few sandwiches or a bread roll, it's worth investigating. The problem won't go away by itself.

But it's not only the gut that can react to gluten. For some people gluten triggers excessive production of chemicals called *cytokines*. These cause inflammation, especially in the brain. High levels of cytokines get seen in people suffering from conditions such as:

- Autism
- Multiple sclerosis
- Alzheimer's disease
- Lou Gehrig's disease
- Parkinson's disease.

I've read a number of case studies where people suffering from some of those conditions have had their symptoms dramatically reduced, or even cleared up altogether, by eliminating grain products from their diet.

Even when the disease appears to have been the result of a cumulative process over years (like the last three listed), when the patients stopped adding more gluten into their system their bodies started to heal themselves – lowering cytokine levels, reducing inflammation in the brain and improving many of their symptoms.

There are a lot of **vegetables and fruits** on the market to choose from. Even a committed carnivore like me will admit that they have an important part to play in a good balanced diet. They provide vitamins, minerals (not as much as they used to – more on that later) and fibre.

The term 'fibre' refers to particular carbohydrates that the body can't break down or absorb. It helps digestion by slowing down the food as it moves through the digestive system and bowel, so the good stuff (like nutrients) gets absorbed more effectively.

The down side is that it can cause bloating, cramping and unwanted farting. You may notice that especially if you switch suddenly to foods that have a higher fibre content than what you've been used to. Overloading your system with fibre can cause diarrhea. At the other extreme, if you don't take in enough fluid (notably water) with the fibre you could find yourself constipated.

If you're eating 'high fibre' foods you should:
- introduce them to your diet gradually, not in a sudden rush;
- don't overdo the quantity;
- chew them really well;
- drink water with them.

I'm not going to detail the pros and cons of every vegetable or fruit, but there are some that can be specifically relevant to men.
Broccoli is supposed to be especially good for blokes. Its combination of high vitamin A, vitamin C and folic acid is said to be a useful cocktail for increasing the sperm count.

Whoever is buying it (or picking it) should look for a good dark shade of green (or blue depending on the type) as that indicates a really high level of vitamin C. Don't overcook it or a lot of the good stuff is lost.

It's not uncommon to find that eating broccoli causes problems with gas, from the embarrassing to the outright painful. If you're suffering like that, but like your broc and want to persist with the benefits of it, try following it up with some peppermint tea. A good old-fashioned remedy!

Tomatoes are tricky. On the one hand, they're full of vitamin C and an anti-oxidant called lycopene that seems to inhibit the growth of cancer cells, particularly in the prostate. The amount required may be quite high though – I've seen up to 10 serves of cooked tomato per week recommended, which seems like a lot of tomato sauce even in Australia!

On the other hand, there are blokes out there who don't react well to tomatoes. Some get skin conditions, others suffer attacks of gout from the acid in the fruit. (Yes, tomato is a fruit, not a vegetable. The seeds are on the inside.) If you're getting symptoms like these already, try cutting tomato in all forms out of your diet for a couple of weeks and see if you improve.

What's more, a lot of the commercially made tomato products like sauces and pastes are seriously loaded with extra sweetener. If you're trying to limit the amount of sugar in your diet – and I really recommend you should – take the trouble to make your own tomato sauce etc, or buy it from someone who doesn't add lashings of sugar or corn syrup.

Pomegranate is one of the best fruits around. It's really rich in anti-oxidants and vitamin C. There are studies that have shown it lowering blood pressure and inhibiting plaque formation in the arteries, and reducing inflammation around the prostate.

There's still research to be done on just how wide-spread those benefits are. They may not be true for everybody. But if you like the taste of pomegranate – the fruit or the unsweetened juice – go for it! It 's very unlikely to do you harm and may well be doing you a lot of good.

All of that being said, it's obvious that **different diets work differently for different people**. And by 'diet' I don't mean 'weight management program', I mean 'what you routinely eat'. Allergies, sensitivities, different metabolisms, natural body shape, blood type, even racial characteristics, all can affect the way a body reacts to particular foods, for better or for worse.

There are three reasons why we eat stuff that's not necessary for our health (or even down-right bad for us):

- quick,

- easy,

- we 'like the taste'.

(Some of that last one has more than a bit to do with the sugars and salt that have been added.)

So take a cooking class. Learn what *you* can do that's quick and easy. Throwing a decent steak on the barbie or in the frypan is a lot better for you than microwaving a meal full of 'processed meat'.

Have a long talk to whoever cooks your dinner if you don't do it yourself.

Look hard at whatever takeaways or dine-out foods you're regularly relying on.

If your lunch comes from the food court in the shopping centre, will a plate of roast beef and veggies really take longer to prepare or eat than a hamburger and fries?

No matter how "good for me" a particular food is touted as being, if I don't like the taste of it I'm going to find excuses not to eat it for long. That said, be prepared to give something a fair go. I've long avoided squash but a friend recently gave me a recipe for lightly frying slices of it in a little good quality butter with pine nuts, shallots and a dash of lemon. It won me over!

On the other side of the coin, there are some foods we love that are bloody hard to give up no matter how "bad for us" they are. Some of that is habit and some of it is probably sugar addiction (even if we don't realise how high the sugar content truly is). But if you've been crazy about fried chicken or snack crackers or chocolate biscuits for forty years it's probably not likely you can just quit them overnight.

So don't, unless you really are one bucket of wings and a potato chip away from a coronary. But cut down. A handful of crackers instead of a boxful at a sitting. Fast food burger once a week (or once a month!) instead of every day. Be realistic.

> **Simply put:** there are certain things that our bodies need to function properly, and others that get in the way of that. The right diet for you is the one you can sustain that has a lot more of the good stuff than the bad.

5.2 You are what you eat: Supplements

I've made the point earlier in the book that over time it's inevitable that a body will wear out. The big problem we face now is accelerated ageing.

The map of chemical reactions happening inside one of your body's cells looks like a map of every single rail network in every major city in the world, all overlaid on each other. It's complicated, and it's fragile. If the natural process of cell regeneration gets compromised, say for instance by the body not getting enough essential nutrients, then the whole framework starts to fall apart.

Energy levels drop, various aspects of health get worse, there's a greater tendency to get sick – you're ageing faster.

Like I said earlier, we should be getting all the nutrients and stuff that we need from the food we eat. There's a problem, though. The food we get to eat these days is not of the same standard that was around years ago.

It starts with the topsoil – that thin bit of dirt that provides most of the minerals and nutrients in the plants we eat, and that feed the animals we eat.

It's thin and getting thinner. In the US topsoil is eroding ten times faster than it's being replenished (which happens by the breakdown of organic material). In places like Africa, India and China it's more like thirty or forty times faster. I've seen one estimate that we've got less than 50 years worth of topsoil left. Globally. That might not directly affect those of us over fifty ourselves, but it's still not a happy thought.

As well as the amount of soil declining, its quality is also on the slide.

A 2006 study determined that during the 20th century, the mineral content of agricultural soil declined by:

- 85% in the USA and Canada,
- 76% in Asia and South America, and
- 74% in Africa, Europe and Australia.

If the soil is starving, then so are the crops it's trying to sustain.

I'm going to quote some figures that are over 25 years old.

Between 1930 and 1987, testing of US crops revealed dramatic declines in some of the essential stuff that we assume we're getting from them:

CROP	RATE of DECLINE	VITAMIN/ MINERAL	SOME OF WHAT IT'S GOOD FOR
Potato	Down 40%	Potassium	Cell function, lowering blood pressure, building muscle mass.
Carrot	Down 75%	Magnesium	Bone formation, glucose metabolism, heart health.
Tomato	Down 90%	Copper	Fighting infection, producing energy.
Cauliflower	Down 50%	Vitamin C	Antioxidant, cell protection, wound healing.
Broccoli & other greens	Down 50%	Vitamin A	Good vision, healthy immune system, cell growth.

It hasn't gotten better in the decades since that table was compiled. Between 1949 and 1999 Canadian spuds lost 57% of their vitamin C and iron, 28% of its calcium, 50% of its riboflavin and 18% of its niacin. British figures for the same period are pretty much the same.

Some of it's in the breeding, believe it or not. The standards set by the US Department of Agriculture are limited to size, shape and colour. They're focused on commercial questions, not consumers' health. Nutritional value doesn't get a look-in. So, because it's regarded as more important that crops look nice and deliver high yields a lot of good stuff has simply been bred out along the way.

I know one grower who spent years selectively breeding chilli peppers for size and shape to fit as many as possible neatly in the jars he preserved and sold them in. Then he wondered why his customers were complaining that they "didn't taste anywhere near as good as they used to." Less heat and less flavour, but they *looked* just right.

Another problem is over-cultivation. Way back when we were a species of wandering hunter-gatherers, we'd cultivate an area for a while, then move on because the people and animals were getting sick because the food wasn't so good any more. Other people would come along and grow different stuff, or other critters would come along and replenish the soil by dropping dung on it and dying on it.

We don't do that any more. We can't. It's hard to move to greener pastures when there aren't any left. We farm the same bits of dirt over and over and over, trying to cram more on and drag more out of it. An acre of corn in the US in 1930 yielded about 50 bushels. By 1960 it was 200 bushels per acre – way more than the soil could sustain.

Sure, we pump it full of NPK fertilizers (nitrate, phosphate and potassium). Useful in the short term, but it makes the soil acidic, killing off the good bacteria and fungi that actually help the plants absorb nutrients. The fertilizers also reduce the availability of other important minerals, for example by affecting selenium so that it can't be taken up by plant roots any more.

Add to that the poisons making their way into our food. Some of it's obvious – the pollution of water that the food absorbs, the chemical sprays and additives that go into and onto fruit, vegies, meat and fish.

Other stuff is less obvious. How many women take The Pill? At least some of the drugs and hormones go into their urine, which goes into the water. This is stuff that sewerage treatment plants aren't designed to filter out so it goes out into the environment. The global environment.

The same goes for toxic stuff like parabens and sodium lauryl sulfates found in shampoos, soaps and such. It's in our food, and it's not healthy.

All of which means that there's a good argument that we need to supplement our diet, however good it is.

"One cannot think well, love well or sleep well if one has not dined well."

- Virginia Woolf

English author 1882 - 1941

There are literally hundreds of nutritional and vitamin supplements on the market. Some products are very specific – a particular vitamin or mineral for instance – others are more 'broad brush' in their approach. Often labeled as a multivitamin or just "multi", a product like this is supposed to plug several of the nutritional gaps we all now face.

In Chapter 6 I'll go into some more detail as to how well or otherwise some of this stuff actually works. But as a general principle I'm happy to state that we will battle to 'eat as well' as past generations did, and if we want to look after our health we need to consume something that makes up for the stuff that's not in our food that our body needs.

They can be the fuel additives that enhance engine performance when the petrol isn't as clean or as potent as you'd like it to be.

> **Simply put**: food is just not as good as it used to be. Nowadays we need more.

5.3 Drugs and alcohol – the poisons we love

I shouldn't need to say a lot about **smoking** being a health hazard. Unless you've been living under a rock for the last twenty years you'll have seen at least some of the advertisements and warnings: graphic pictures of clogged arteries, decaying lungs, damaged hearts etc. I *will* give you some figures in a bit.

Neither am I going to trot out "research" that's been paid for by some tobacco company saying (like in a 1950's magazine ad I saw recently) Doctor Jones of XYZ Medical Centre says, "smoking is good for you".

I've known people who smoked well into their 80s or later. Maybe if they didn't smoke they'd have lived beyond 120, but I doubt it. On the other hand though, I knew a girl who died of lung cancer at age 25 – the closest she'd come to a cigarette was sitting opposite a chain smoker on the bus home from work.

My thought is that it's a gamble. I reckon we've all got something like a switch in our bodies that 'turns on' a cancer. A genetic predisposition, if you want to be technical.

Genetics don't cause disease. They're a blueprint within your body – something has to activate them. You can be born with a proclivity to a disease (cancer, heart disease, maybe even depression) that gives you a 'hair trigger' compared to other people, but something has to set it off. Conversely you might have a genetic 'resistance' to certain conditions that makes the 'switch' hard to turn on, like the long-lived smokers.

But the odds don't look to be in favour of the smokers. Let's face it, the chemicals being inhaled are toxic.

"It is now proved beyond doubt that smoking is one of the leading causes of statistics."

- Fletcher Knebel

U.S. writer 1911 - 1993

A National Health Survey in Australia in 2008 found that heart disease and stroke were more common in adults who'd smoked at some time in their life (8%) than those who'd never touched a ciggie (5%). 'That's not too bad,' I thought.

Then I read the lung-related figures.

A smoker or ex-smoker was 1.6 times as likely to have bronchitis as a non-smoker.

They were 6 times more likely to have emphysema than non-smokers.

And then, there's lung cancer. The World Health Organisation in 2009 issued a Report on the Global Tobacco Epidemic, in which they reckoned that "the role of smoking in increasing the chance of lung cancer is one of the most widely known of tobacco's harmful effects on human health".

Interesting that they say 'increasing the chance of' – not 'causing'. That reinforces what I said about it being a gamble.

Here are some figures on lung cancer death rates in Australia since the Second World War:

GENDER	YEAR	DEATHS PER 100,000 AGED > 15
Male	1945	11.3
Male	1985	74.8
Male	2008	59.0
Female	1945	3.5
Female	1985	22.0
Female	2008	33.4

Some of that rise may be because since 1945 doctors have gotten better at diagnosing lung cancer. I know in the 50's I had an uncle whose cause of death was listed as "bad cough". It might also be that other potentially fatal diseases are being treated better, so the lung cancer now has time to develop to the point of being a killer.

But I suspect it's no coincidence that the drop in men's death rates between 1985 and 2008 reflects a noticeable drop in the number of male smokers in that time. In 1989 31% of men were 'current' smokers, and 38% had never smoked. By 2008 only 23% were smoking and 47% were 'never'.

The rates in women didn't fall nearly as much. 24% 'current' smokers in 1989 went down to 19% in 2008. The percentage of women who 'never smoked' didn't improve at all, staying at 58%.

It's a stress reliever for some, I get that. Some of the 4,000 chemicals in a smoke can be relaxing, even though they raise the heart rate and blood pressure. In 2008, 31% of Australians who said they had high levels of stress were daily smokers, and 63% had been regular smokers at some point in their lives. If it helps you so much that you're willing to take the gamble, then that's your right to choose. You know the risks and the potential damage.

If you're lucky enough to be one of the resistant ones, I'm happy for you. But there's only one way to find that you're not, and the consequences are dramatic. I admit, I decided not to bet my life.

For many of us, there's a lot to like about **alcohol**. It's a big part of the social life of a lot of blokes. It's got friends in high places – the Apostle Paul said that wine is good for us, and Benjamin Franklin said that beer is proof that God loves us and wants us to be happy!

"There are better things in the world than alcohol, but alcohol sort of compensates for not getting them."
- Terry Pratchett
British author 1948 - 2015

The part of alcohol that works on our brains is ethanol. When you drink it goes from your intestines straight to your bloodstream. From there it goes, among other places, to the brain – and that's where it gets interesting.

Ethanol is classed as a 'central nervous system depressant'. "But wait a minute," you say. "Alcohol doesn't depress me – it puts me in the mood to party!"

Yep. Because what ethanol depresses is a neurotransmitter in your brain (*glutamate* if you want to know the detail) that normally excites neurons. The brain is slower to respond to stimuli, and less likely to recognise the 'controls' that normally stop you from dancing on the table, trying to chat up the hot bird with the gigantic boyfriend, or driving home when you can hardly stand.

It activates a particular acid in your brain (the powerfully named *gamma aminobutyric acid* or GABA) that makes you feel calm and sleepy, while it also triggers the release of dopamine, which tends to make you feel good but can also make you sleepy.

It's a complicated set of reactions, and because everyone's body chemistry is a little bit different (even one person's can change according to what they've eaten or done that day!) there is no hard-and-fast rule about how one particular bloke will react to a certain number of beers on any given day.

If you knock back a serious lot of the stuff though, it's a safe bet that the effect won't be good. Flooding the brain – four bottles of wine, a bottle-and-a-bit of spirits, a dozen-plus stubbies in a session – can depress your brain function so much that it fails to do its job properly. Critical things like keeping your heart beating and reminding you to breathe.

That last one explains why some people die of "alcohol poisoning". They pass out and their brain doesn't remind the body to breathe. Alternatively, their gag reflex is suppressed by the alcohol, so when they throw up nothing stops them from inhaling the vomit and they drown in it. Vale Bon Scott, the real voice of AC/DC.

But alcohol's effect on your body isn't usually that catastrophic that quickly.

Your liver metabolises alcohol at the rate of about 29 ml (1 fluid ounce) per hour, but it gets knocked around in the process, not least by the sugars that are integral to alcohol. Think back to Chapter 5.1 – excess sugar (glucose) becomes fat. If your doctor warns you about "fatty liver" it's a good bet that somewhere in that conversation you'll be asked about your drinking habits!

Add to that the fact that your kidney gets knocked around every time it passes out the waste products – the bigger the binge, the more toxins, the more damage.

Alcohol can be fun. It can also damage you, and that damage can accumulate and become more obvious the older you get. One of the ironic aspects of this is that among the most common and most obvious effects is that you find you "can't drink like you used to."

> **Simply put:** the more moderate your alcohol consumption, the less damage you do to your brain and other vital organs, in both short- and long-term.

Let's face it, **drugs** in general are designed to affect your body or brain in some way by messing with your chemistry. If they're prescription or 'over-the-counter' drugs, taken in the right dose they're supposed to help.

To heal if you're lucky, but at least to ease some symptoms. It might be by triggering or halting the production of some chemicals, for instance to dull some transmissions along nerves. Some pain killers work that way.

'Performance enhancing' drugs tend to mimic your own hormones, boosting strength or endurance in the way things like testosterone and adrenalin do.

And then there are the 'recreational drugs'. Uppers, downers, whatever, their effect is to mess with the chemistry of your brain. That's a tricky business because the brain is just so bloody complicated. (If your brain was so simple that you could understand it, you'd be too simple understand it.)

Three people can share the same joint and have three different reactions. Their body chemistry is different. Move up to drugs that are a lot more potent and the differences can be more pronounced. One guy gets happy, one gets morose, another turns violent and another falls asleep. Maybe another one dies.

There isn't a set figure that defines where 'overdose' starts. Some heroin users last for years, others for weeks.

I go back to the analogy of that finely tuned car you got on your seventeenth birthday. Pump some crazy souped-up rocket fuel into it and it might just go like a bat out of hell for a while (if it doesn't immediately blow up) – but it's not what the engine was built for and it won't last.

96

5.4 Exercise. Don't just sit there – move something!

Any exercise is better than none.

In this little section I'm going to talk about the guys that are already stirring their stumps on a reasonably regular basis. Someone whose idea of weightlifting is hauling himself out of bed in the morning is hereby advised to go read Chapter 6.3.

If you're a young bloke who's already getting regular exercise then good on you. You're giving yourself the best chance you can. If you're a not-so-young bloke who's getting regular exercise then even better. You're protecting your insides *and* the stuff that keeps them all together.

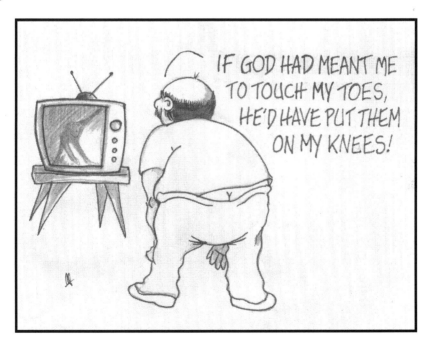

"Even if you're on the right track, you'll get run over if you just sit there."

- The Positive Life Store

I mentioned earlier the importance of muscle mass. It's not just about strength, it's about recovery from injury, illness, surgery etc. That's because your muscle tissue acts as a reservoir for proteins and other chemicals that get released when the body goes into 'recovery mode'.

The best way to protect and improve the state of your muscles is through resistance training (also called strength training). That's exercise that increases muscle strength and endurance. You might use weights or resistance bands. It's been shown to be useful for both the prevention and treatment of sarcopenia (the muscle wasting condition I talked about back in Chapter 3.3).

Resistance training has been reported to do good things for your nerves, your muscles, your hormone production, and even how well you process the protein you consume.

You're also helping your lungs and heart by exercising them, and by working on keeping your body fat down you're helping your liver, too.

It might surprise you to learn that there's good research indicating that physical exercise helps the brain, too.

Al is a good mate of mine who's an enthusiastic long distance runner, and has been for the twenty-plus years I've known him. He recently suffered a serious heart problem – an artery ruptured and he collapsed at the kitchen sink.

He survived, recovered well, and has started running again. I asked whether he'd been overdoing it, and if the running had been putting too much strain on his heart in the first place. Al replied that he'd asked the doctor the same thing. The answer was that no, the rupture literally could have happened to anyone, and that the overall fitness he had from years of exercise was what actually enabled him to survive. If it had been me, I wouldn't be writing this now.

> **Simply put:** regular moderate exercise is good for your body, short term and long term.

5.5 Armour up!

If you value your car or bike, you keep it clean and polished, right? It's not about showing off (although we ought to admit that sometimes comes into it) – it's about making the machine last longer. Keep the rust out.

The same applies to your body. It's not 'girly' to look after your skin. You don't have to be 'metrosexual' or a glam rock wannabe to put stuff on your face.

I'm not talking about make-up, or cosmetics. I'm talking about skin care. Moisturiser, toner, hydrating lotions – that sort of thing.

It baffles me that there's such a big gap between the multi-million dollar industry that is women's skin care and what's available for blokes. We've got the same skin, which faces the same problems (pardon the pun), yet we have a fraction of the range to choose from. If you take shaving cream and aftershave out of the picture the gap gets *really* huge.

The same skin, made up of the same cells, with the same challenges (sun, wind, pollution, toxins we consume) should get the same solution, shouldn't it? Luckily there *are* some products out there that work well on blokes without making us look or feel 'pretty'.

Having your complexion looking the best it can may or may not matter to you. You might be past caring about your schoolboyish charm. But protecting and strengthening your skin is a different matter.

Get the grime and dirt and crap cleaned off. The longer they stay on your skin the more toxins find their way into your system.

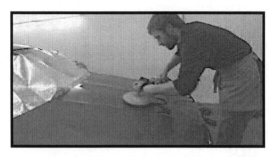

Keep the skin moisturized and toned. Not because it feels nice when your partner strokes it (okay, that can be a bonus!), but because the cells below the surface are really your body's first line of defence against airborne disease and bacteria. The plumper and healthier those cells are, the stronger your system is.

Cleaning isn't as easy as it might seem. Soaps, gels and cleansers will (usually) get the dirt off the surface – sometimes by scraping that surface off – but a lot of them are loaded with chemicals that may in the long run be just as bad for you.

The same applies to toners, moisturisers, shaving creams – anything you rub on your skin. Better than 60% of what's applied on the outside gets absorbed all the way into the bloodstream and so gets into your liver, heart, brain, gut etc.

Some of the chemicals all-too-commonly used have been proven dangerous, some haven't been around long enough to "prove" what long-term cumulative damage they're doing but have evidence stacking up against them. Read the label! Here's a list of ingredients to be wary of:
- Parabens (increasingly found in cancer tumours)
- Sodium laurel sulfates (make lather, used in industrial cleaners, irritate skin)
- Formaldehyde-releasing preservatives (cancer causing) e.g.:
    Formalin
    Morbicid acid
    Methyline Oxide
    Methylene Glycol
    DMDM hydantoin
    Diazolidinyl urea

- Butylated hydroxyanisole BHA
- Butylated hydroxytoluene BHT (both endocrine & hormone disruptors)
- Triclosan (skin irritant & hormone disruption)
- DEA (makes foam - high doses or frequent use linked to cancer)

If you reckon that list is ugly, what they're doing under the top layer of your skin is probably uglier! The trouble is, a lot of these chemicals get pushed out onto supermarket shelves too quickly, without their long-term effects being properly tested or understood. There's less care about the real safety of a product than there is about how it looks.

An attractive colour or a rich thick foam that looks great in an ad (so you think it *must* work better) is more important than the possibility that putting it on your skin every day may make you sterile, or even eventually kill you.   Just think – you could be the best-looking corpse in the cemetery!

The other important bit of skin care every bloke should do is protection against the sun. The 'bronzed Aussie' tan might look great but the surgery scars after melanoma removal don't.

Fifty years ago there might have been an excuse. Most people had never heard of a "basal cell carcinoma". I had a neighbour who prided himself on being "brown as a bloody berry". He worked outside all day, wore a hat because he didn't like getting his nose burnt, always wore shorts and nearly always was without a shirt by ten in the morning. He died of skin cancer in his fifties.

My Dad was a similar case study. Overalls during the week, but his weekend 'uniform' was shorts and a blue singlet. Skin cancer didn't claim him, but judging by the tumour removed from his forehead it probably would have if throat cancer hadn't got there first.

It's not hard. Put a decent quality sunscreen on any bits that aren't covered by a hat, shirt, shorts or trousers. That includes your feet and hands. Every sunburn, whether it reaches the point of being painful or not, brings you one step closer to hearing the words, "I'm afraid we're going to have to operate to cut that out, sir." I know – I've got my own scars to prove it.

Look for a sunscreen that's not greasy and won't block your pores, especially if you're using it often.

Polishing the car doesn't really make it go faster or run better, but it does help it last longer!

Simply put: your skin protects you. You should protect it.

5.6 The air that we breathe

You can't see air. That's the theory. Good theory. Have you seen the air above Sydney on a bad day, or Chicago or London? Or perhaps worst of all, Beijing?

There's a good chance you've at least seen pictures of any or all of the above. They're not pretty, although they make sunrise and sunset look dramatic. Seen in 'real life' those bad day skies are even worse, believe me. For one thing, my eyes were itching so much that seeing *anything* was a challenge.

The eyes don't like it and the lungs like it less. Coughing. Wheezing. Choking. A cocktail of chemicals making breathing a challenge.

High on the list is the exhaust fume carbon monoxide, that popular suicide choice when concentrated through a hosepipe. There are plenty of other toxic chemicals and heavy metals up there too, not just the ones being pumped out by motor vehicles.

The cities I mentioned are just well-recognised offenders. They're hardly unique. The more industrialised the area, the worse the cocktail, but even in less developed areas the air cops contaminants from various sources. Smoke from cooking and heating fires, methane gas from quantities of farm animals. (It's estimated that about 12% of all the methane going into Australia's atmosphere comes from the belches and farts of livestock.) Tiny particles, microscopic even, which get into the lungs and the blood, block things up and ultimately stress lots of your body's systems.

Here's a cheerless thought. If you live in a city it's likely that the air inside your home is even more polluted than the air outside. That's because the air in your home contains all the same noxious fumes you'll find outside (after all, that's where the air comes from) but it's also contaminated with volatile organic compounds (VOCs). These VOCs are there because you put them there. They come from paint, adhesives, chemical cleaners, bug spray, air fresheners, and anything else you spray into the air in your home.

These products are filling the air in your place, and therefore your lungs, with yet more toxins.

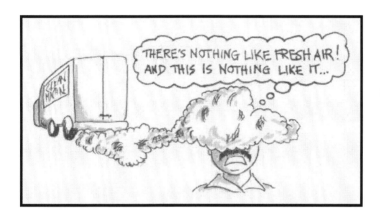

The best solution to that particular problem is to control or eliminate the sources of the indoor pollutants. Use natural products when you can. Pump packs instead of aerosols. Don't hold the button down on the can for quite as long.

If the air outside your home is at least reasonably clean (i.e. it doesn't go brown on bad days) then make certain the place has adequate ventilation. Open a few windows whenever you get the chance. Otherwise, choosing a quality air filter or purifier is an option.

When possible, get as far away as you can from the most polluted environment for as long as you can. Take a holiday for a couple of weeks in the country. Spend a weekend at the beach, especially if it's a quiet one without a busy city attached. Go for a walk in a park at lunchtime or after work - one that has plenty of trees. Plants are great air filters, even if we are asking a lot of them these days.

> **Simply put:** breathing is essential, so inhale the best air you can whenever you can.

5.7 Surviving stress

There's a vicious cycle inside the body when it comes to **stress**. It probably goes all the way back to caveman days.

Tension in the muscles signals 'danger' to the brain. That switches on a 'fight or flight' response (or one of the other Fs - see Chapter 4.4) which is great if you're faced with a sabre-tooth tiger but not so helpful when you're stressed by another aggravating e-mail from Head Office.

The stress response:

- Raises blood pressure
- Releases stored fats and sugars into the system for energy (where they don't all get used and the leftovers become toxins)
- Shuts down the digestive system (it's hard for the body to concentrate on digesting properly if you're running away from big teeth and claws)
- Reduces sex drive (see the comment about digestion above)
- Can cause panic attacks.

All that stuff starts to happen, and you get stressed about how bad you feel, because you haven't actually fought or fled from a real danger. Your body and brain get confused and it all gets worse. Like I mentioned back in Chapter 4.4, it gets even more difficult when the absence of 'fight' nor 'flight' options stays unresolved for any length of time.

If you start to feel overwhelmed, try putting these steps into practice. I won't call them 'simple steps' because I know very often they're not. But remember: it's *your* life and if you won't be your own mate, who will?

Don't overextend yourself.

Know your limits and stick to them. Refuse to accept added responsibilities when you feel as if you're taking on too much. Always remember that it's okay to say "no."

Tackle tasks one step at a time. Don't get ahead of yourself. That's like trying to tile the roof before the foundation is laid or the walls are up.

> # "When the 'big picture' makes you drop your head, then think about small goals. Chunk it up."
>
> *- Lleyton Hewitt*
>
> 80 weeks ranked as world #1 tennis player

Avoid people who stress you out.

If someone consistently causes stress in your life and you can't turn the relationship around, limit the amount of time you spend with that person or end the relationship entirely. If you're dealing with a difficult family member, be honest and up front with them about why you're distancing yourself from the relationship. You might even find that speaking your mind and letting others know how you feel will actually improve your relationship with them. That should reduce your stress even further.

And remember, if they get all tetchy and upset, it's become their problem, not yours. They have to deal with your honesty.

Take control of your environment.

If the evening news makes you anxious or gets you angry, turn the TV off. If your commute makes you irritable or nervous, think about the route you're taking and allow yourself sufficient time to reach your destination safely and on time without feeling rushed. Maybe you leave earlier, or find a way to be comfortable about arriving later. Or work out a different way to travel.

If you find that large crowds add to your anxiety, stay away from crowded footpaths, congested stores or shopping malls during peak hours.

Avoid sensitive topics.

If you get upset over religion, politics, or other hot-button issues, cross them off your conversation list. If someone else starts on about something that fires you up, smile, nod, and walk away. Go do something else and don't play their game.

A bloke who is in a long-term relationship (marriage or whatever else) can be, or at least seem, more vulnerable to stress. Stress is a powerful thing, and small problems in a relationship can become exaggerated when either partner takes their personal stresses out on the other. The stress snowballs and the results of the behavior can be devastating.

If you're With Someone and you want to avoid stress coming between you, here are some more steps you might want to consider, further to the ones I listed above.

Take time to decompress.

After a stressful day at work, many people (male *and* female) need time alone to decompress before they're ready to talk. And a conversation you have to force yourself or the other person to have is never a good thing. Allow yourselves a few minutes. Get over the day and get your bearings straight. Watch some television, read a few pages of your favorite book, or even sit outside and catch some sunshine if the weather permits. At the very least, take a few deep breaths.

Teamwork: work with each other.

Being in a relationship is like being on a team. For the team to be successful, you need to support each other. Communicate and talk about the details of your day. Sharing your feelings can help strengthen the partnership. If your feelings are out in the open, you'll be less likely to "blow up" and take the day's stresses out on each other. Listen to each other. Talk *with* your partner, not *at* them. Do the best you can to be positive and supportive. Don't make it a competition to see who's had the worst day!

Don't point the finger.

When we're stressed we often default to taking it out on the first available, or easiest target. Unfortunately your partner is frequently the most available target when you're stressed. It might be blame, or it might just be dumping the day's crap. Breathe. Try to see things from your partner's point of view. If you can see where the other person is coming from, that will increase your understanding of the situation. Don't assume that you're the one who has all the problems, *or* all the answers.

> **Simply put:** stress happens but there are things you
> can do to ease the effects.

5.8 ~~Body~~ brain building

I made it clear (I hope) back in Chapter 3.7 that although neurons do die off with ageing, in a healthy brain that rate is only gradual. And that while the dead cells don't seem to be replaced, the living healthy neurons can continue to grow new axons. Making new pathways. Learning new things.

So, what's the trick to that?

Exercise, of the mental variety. Do stuff you don't regularly do. Here are a few ideas:

- Read new books, not just reread the same couple of favourites over and over.

- Do the crossword in the paper – even if you don't finish, look at the answers next day.

- Try a jigsaw – blow a dollar or two at the Op Shop so if you don't like it you can give it back.

- Watch – really *watch*, not just use it as background noise – some different TV, maybe a documentary or two.

- Go to a regular trivia night at the pub or wherever. So what if you don't win? You might learn some fun new stuff, and discover you actually know more than you thought!

- You don't like academic stuff. You just like watching the footy. How well do you know the rules? Try learning to be a coach, or a ref – junior clubs are crying out for the help!

- Teach someone else how to do something you reckon you know well.

- Find different ways of getting to work, or the pub, or the shops. Who knows what you'll see on some of those back streets?

You get the picture? It's about doing things that are different to your routine. That's what makes your brain rewire itself. Doing the same stuff over and over has the same effect on the brain as repeatedly driving a cart along the same dirt road: eventually you get stuck in a rut.

If you haven't been flexing the mental muscles enough, as you get older you'll start to see the signs. Or else, other people will, even if you don't.

The people at the National Dementia Helpline have put together a "Memory Concerns Checklist". Have a read through and score yourself (honestly!). Circle **R**arely, **S**ometimes or **O**ften beside each statement.

- I have trouble remembering events that happened recently. R S O

- I have trouble finding the right word. R S O

- I have trouble remembering the day and date. R S O

- I forget where things are usually kept. R S O

- I have difficulty adjusting to any changes in my daily routine. R S O

- I have trouble understanding magazine or newspaper articles, or following a story in a book or on TV. R S O

- I find it hard to follow conversations, especially in groups. R S O

- I have problems handling financial matters such as banking or calculating change. R S O

- I have difficulty with everyday activities such as remembering how long between visits from family or friends, or cooking a meal I've always cooked well. R S O

- I am losing interest in activities I'd normally enjoy. R S O

- I have difficulties thinking through problems. R S O

- Family or friends have commented about my poor memory. R S O

A couple of 'Sometimes' is okay. A bunch of them isn't. 'Often' isn't good at all. The more you've answered 'Often', the more important it is that you talk to a doctor. It doesn't necessarily mean you have dementia, or are on the way to it – there are quite a few possible causes. But major changes in memory aren't normal at any age and should be taken seriously.

Simply put: if you're aware that your memory is getting worse, don't ignore it. Talk to your doctor (before you forget!).

.o0o.

6 WHAT CAN A BLOKE DO?

"Ah, mate," you say, "All that stuff - that's just getting older. Nothing you can do about that."

Right enough, like I said last chapter there's only one cure for getting older, and that's dying.

But I reckon there are plenty of ways to manage the effects.

Chapter 5 was about prevention. This one is about finding ways of getting better.

> **"To get back my youth I would do anything in the world, except take exercise, get up early, or be respectable."**
>
> *- Oscar Wilde*
>
> Irish author and playwright

I've talked to a lot of people with a lot of different ideas. I found people who are really, *really* good in their fields. I've talked to doctors who specialise in different things, scientists, Eastern medicine people – all sides of the medical profession. I've spoken to people who are experts in other disciplines – martial arts, yoga, alternative therapies.

I've put together what I reckon are the best answers and suggestions that I've been given. I'm not going to say, "This one's right and that one's wrong," because what *I* think or say might not be true for *you*.

You know that weird thing you find in some clothes stores – "One size fits all". What a load of crap that is!

I can see me going into a shop with my mates Gav and Chris, and the three of us trying on some 'one size fits all' items. Yeah, right. A shirt that may be okay for me – Gav might squeeze into it but if he sneezes the buttons are going to fly off and drill holes in the wall. Chris tries on the track pants that were snug but okay on Gav, and realises he can get both of his legs down one leg of the pants. Technically speaking they might fit, but they're sure not a *good* fit.

Likewise with health 'solutions'. There are a huge number of things that make us all different. Different in body – your family background, your level of fitness, body shape, history (accidents etc.), allergies, food preferences. Different in mind – your experiences, memories, upbringing, biases for and against, likes and dislikes.

Doctors are taught to diagnose a patient using something called 'the standard medical procedure':

- Get a proper history (i.e. a lot more than "why are you here today?");

- do an examination, don't just assume the patient is describing or explaining everything you need to know;

- carry out investigation on problem area(s). That means tests: blood tests, MRI, x-ray or whatever is appropriate.

That last one is there to make the crucial step from symptom to cause. It means going beyond sympathetically chalking up your problem to "just getting older".

As a plan of attack for any health professional, whatever their field, 'conventional' or otherwise, it can't be beat.

Different therapists have different opinions. That's okay, but it bothers me that there are some who still don't accept that male menopause even exists. I read a quote from someone at the University of Rhode Island declaring that: "Men can't have menopause because they don't have ovaries." By now you should know it's a lot more complicated than that.

Okay, so recognising that different things work for different people, here's a range of stuff I've learned. Take a look around the shop, as it were. If one person's ideas don't appeal, or seem too weird or just plain wrong, or you've tried it and it didn't work (assuming you gave it a *decent* go and didn't just make a half-assed effort to keep someone else off your back) – then look at something else, until you find something that *does* work for you.

Remember too that a bad therapist doesn't mean that the therapy itself is bad. I've met some GPs who have been pretty lousy: disinterested, poor communication skills, not up to date with treatments. But that doesn't mean I'll never go to another doctor. The same goes for chiropractors, yoga teachers or whoever else offers a service you might try.

> **Simply put:** there is no one right answer. Keep an open mind and find what works best for you.

6.1 Conventional "Western" medicine

Your regular GP is a good place to start, assuming that you've already got one and have a good open trusting relationship with him/her.

The British National Health Service suggests that anxiety/stress based symptoms are best treated by a combination of medication, exercise, relaxation and what they call 'cognitive behavioural therapy'. That last doozy pretty much means 'talking to someone'.

> ## "Men are often in denial about their symptoms, they have this 'it will get better' attitude... ignorance and denial can be a dangerous combination. It is important that men explain their symptoms properly to their doctor."
> *- Dr. Michael Gillman*
> Brisbane-based men's health specialist

You have to be confident you're talking to someone who is taking you seriously.

I've spent a lot of words in this book explaining that there are a lot of factors influencing your physical and mental health as you get older beyond just "ageing". There are a *lot* of treatments out there, and many if not most are very specific to very specific problems, for example:

- Angina tablets
- Anti-depressants
- Arthritis treatments
- Aspirin for heart conditions...

See? I haven't even got past the letter A!

One for the middle-aged bloke that gets argued about a lot (the treatment, not the bloke) is **testosterone therapy**. The thinking goes: that's what's declining, so if we ramp it back up that will fix things.

Some doctors think it's a bad idea. Others reckon it's a good idea. Some say it's not likely to do either much harm or much good!

The Victorian government's Betterhealth website reckons:

> "The effects of testosterone replacement therapy in men are currently being studied, including possible risks such as prostate cancer. Of concern are several recent studies suggesting a rise in cardiovascular disease after commencement of testosterone therapy in older men."

Then I go to another medical website that tells me:

> "Contrary to fears of the potential adverse effects of testosterone on cardiovascular disease, there are over forty epidemiological studies which have examined the relationship of testosterone levels to the presence or development of coronary heart disease, and none have shown a positive correlation. Many of these studies have found the presence of coronary disease to be associated with low testosterone levels."

The Drug Therapeutics Bulletin warns:

> "Testosterone therapy may not be effective in treating male menopause, and may raise the risk of urinary tract blockage and prostate cancer."

Another website, another view:

> "Cross-sectional studies have not shown raised testosterone levels at the time of diagnosis of prostate cancer, and in fact, low testosterone at the time of diagnosis has been linked with more locally aggressive and malignant tumors. This may reflect loss of hormone related control of the tumor or the effect of a more aggressive tumor in decreasing testosterone levels."

David Handelsman, MD, PhD, professor and director of the ANZAC Research Institute at the University of Sydney says:

> "older men with low testosterone levels do not need testosterone therapy unless they have diseases of their pituitary or testes."

Dr. Gerald Lewis is a leading New Zealand cardiologist. His view is that testosterone levels have a normal, natural rate of decline. He told me:

> "Your doctor can do a test to determine whether yours is significantly lower than it should be for your age. If it is, and *only if it is significantly low*, then the application of something like a testosterone cream should be enough. Don't use it if you don't really need it! You risk over-elevating your testosterone. That can, and probably will cause behavioural changes, and not for the better."

Where does all that leave us? Besides confused?

If your doctor reckons it will help, and you're okay with the idea – give it a try. But be aware of what's going on with your body. Are you feeling better? Are you getting any side effects?

One mate of mine who tried testosterone treatment in the form of HRT injections suddenly developed really bad sleep apnoea. He snored like a sawmill (which didn't please his partner), and it quickly got to the point where he'd stop breathing while asleep. That's not a common reaction, apparently, but the point is to be aware of *any* changes.

I've got another mate who moved from injections to using a testosterone cream. He's been on it for years and he swears by it. Yet I've read complaints from guys who reckon the cream made them break out in a rash.

It may well be that your particular symptoms are coming from other causes that should be treated first.

Dr. A. R. Marin of the Sanoviv Medical Institute was really emphatic about this when I talked to him.

> "HRT is *not* the first line of treatment. It can actually make symptoms worse if there's a different underlying cause, so a patient having HRT *must* have constant regular monitoring by their doctor."

You may not need testosterone therapy if you can get any 'different underlying causes' sorted out first. The key is for your doctor to test you thoroughly, not just take what they think may be an easy option. You can help by asking questions – if you don't understand the answers get them to try again. If you're still not happy, look elsewhere.

Simply put: there are arguments for and against **testosterone therapy. If it's recommended for you then try it, but** *you* **decide whether it's doing you harm or good.**

I was talking with my gastrologist (a good bloke named Angus Thomson) about **'detox' programs**. We agreed that, unless the situation was really dire and urgent, it was smarter to make the process gradual and steady over a few months rather than a 'crash-through' two day program that you might do once a year (chances are you'll go back to knocking your system around for the other 363 days anyway).

As Angus put it, "When you push nature, nature finds ways of pushing back."

That's not to say, "don't detox". By now I reckon you realise I think we've all got too many toxins in our bodies – some we knowingly put there ourselves and some that we cop from our environment and the stuff we eat.

A short rapid program is a bit like flushing a toilet. The big obvious lumps are gotten rid of – most of the time – but occasionally some persist anyway, and there's usually stuff left clinging to the edges. The longer that crap has been sitting on the porcelain the harder it is to shift the evidence.

I know a bloke who eats and drinks all manner of rubbish almost all year round, and once a year does a 'Rapid Detox' he buys from the supermarket. He doesn't actually read the label and has no idea what's in the product, how it's made or what it's actually doing to his body.

So he loads himself up with sugar, bad fats, chemicals and preservatives for eleven and seven-eighths months, then gulps down a dose of more chemicals that may or may not do more good than harm – then he starts all over again. And wonders why he feels crook so often.

You don't need a 'product' to detox. Some of them might be a handy kickstart, but really your own body knows how to detoxify itself. It just needs time. Stop loading it up with the bad stuff and give yourself a chance to heal.

And to make it really effective, keep as many of those toxins out of your regular diet as possible. That way, when they *do* appear, they're in an amount that your body can manage.

Simply put: it's a good idea to detox. Do it gradually and do it regularly.

Western medicine tends to be less concerned with **cause versus effect**. It often focuses on symptoms more than what's really responsible for them. Plenty of doctors have told me that's how they've always been trained!

A cynic might suggest that if the doctors fix the real problem then they've cut off a steady income. I reckon that's a bit harsh in the majority of cases – I believe most doctors genuinely want to do what's best for their patients. It comes back to their training, and to too few patients actually asking serious questions about their own health.

Here's a tip to help with understanding your doctor: if he/she tells you you've got anything ending with –*itis*, that means inflammation.

- Arthritis: your joints
- Bronchitis: the tubes in your lungs.
- Colitis: your colon.
- Dermatitis: your skin
- Encephalitis: your brain.
- Hepatitis: your liver.
- Rhinitis: the lining of your nose.

You get the picture?

Inflammation can mean redness, warmth, swelling and/or pain, but remember – it's a symptom. You can manage a symptom, but what you really need is to identify and treat the cause.

If your doctor isn't interested in doing more than dealing with the symptoms, I suggest you thank him or her politely, take what they're offering if you're comfortable with it, but go look for a second opinion.

Look for someone who will explore *why* that part of your body is inflamed. Some of these conditions do occur more as we age, but ageing itself isn't a reason. It might be the build-up of particular chemicals in your body. Even ones that aren't 'toxic' can provoke inflammation if you're carrying too much of them or they're reacting to something else in your system, remember.

Among the best habits you can get into (if you haven't already) is getting **regular tests** done. If you already do, then consider your back patted, mate. If not, it's time you started.

I recently read about a bloke who collapsed while on holiday visiting the old Vietcong tunnels in Vietnam. He was lucky – a decent doctor in Ho Chi Minh City spotted that it was a serious problem with his heart. A quick medical evacuation to Sydney (*that's* why travel insurance is important!) and he was having a heart valve replaced.

He'd spent two years figuring that the occasional shortness of breath was just a bit of a flare-up of the asthma he'd had as a kid. He didn't smoke, worked out at the gym three or four times a week, and he was just too bloody busy for a visit to the GP.

That visit, and a decent conversation with his doctor, would probably have meant getting some tests done. The problem would have been spotted so he wouldn't have had the Big Trip ruined or had his life put at risk.

The first time you get a test done is important. It's a picture of where you're at in a particular moment. If there's something wrong you can start to work on it, and if the tests are clear then you can either relax and keep doing what you're doing, or if there are symptoms happening you can cross something off the list and look at another possible cause.

The best thing about having a regular program of tests is that you and your doctor can see patterns and trends. "This is getting worse, we better do something about it." "This is getting better, that treatment or those lifestyle changes are working!"

A few regular tests that I've seen recommended:

- Cholesterol – check at least every five years from the age of 45

- Blood pressure – check every two years, more if you're told it's high or low

- Blood glucose – check every three years from 55, or 45 if you've got a family history of diabetes or you know you're well overweight

- Faecal Occult Blood Test (FOBT) – bowel cancer screening, every two years from the age of 50.

It's your body, your responsibility. It's up to you to keep your eyes on what's happening. Be **self-aware**. Monitor your own symptoms so you know if they're getting worse or better.

One of the perils of whatever therapy you choose to try is that not everyone in the medical profession – whatever path they claim to follow – is totally honest.

Professor Andrew McLachlan, leading pharmacy researcher at the George Institute for Global Health gives two examples. Some over-the-counter analgesics are marketed as targeting pain in specific parts of the body, which he maintains is pharmacologically impossible. He's published a study on acute lower back pain demonstrating that paracetamol doesn't have a substantial impact on reducing either pain or recovery time in people with recent onset lower back pain.

He is also critical of 'alternative' therapists who assert that all their remedies are safe to take alongside conventional medicines simply because they're made from all natural ingredients. He gives the example of the herbal antidepressant St. John's Wort, which increases the rate that warfarin is metabolized. That means there's less of the drug in the patient's body than the dose they think they're on, and that increases their risk of having a stroke.

Some doctors are now arguing *against* what they call "over-prescription" – the tendency to treat every ailment as a 'medical condition' and throw drugs at it. It can mean side-effects that are worse than the original problem, especially if drugs prescribed by different doctors react with each other in unpleasant ways.

Dr. David Le Couteur is a professor at the Sydney University and a specialist at Concord Hospital. He takes the opposite approach. "We undiagnose, we withdraw treatment, and we de-prescribe – and people improve. We do it not to reduce cost. We do it to improve quality and quantity of life."

For many conditions, drugs are not the only answer. They may not be the best answer for you. They may not even be the *right* answer for you. Try what's prescribed for you, sure. But be alert to, and aware of two key things:
- Is the condition improving?
- Are there any signs of side-effects, and if so, how serious are they?

> **Simply put:** Medicine can be an important part of getting you well, but the benefits have to outweigh the negatives, otherwise you're just replacing one problem with another, possibly worse one.

6.1b Sex and the surgery

Worries about sex are often those that most concern a bloke (and get talked about least). I reckon there's a whole new book to be written there, and okay, I will.

Meanwhile, here's some very specific stuff that you could, no, make that *should* talk with your doctor about if you're having trouble getting it up or keeping it up (which are the most common complaints...)

Your doctor is likely to ask you a number of questions. If he or she doesn't, then they're letting you down. It's not nosey, or rude. It's about finding the cause behind the symptom, and that's a good thing! Be prepared to think about and answer questions such as these (from the Mayo Clinic in the USA):

* What other health concerns or chronic conditions do you have?
* Have you had any other sexual problems?
* When did you first begin noticing sexual problems?
* Have you had any changes in sexual *desire*, as distinct from performance?
* Do your erectile problems occur only sometimes, often or all of the time?
* Do you get erections during masturbation, with a partner or while you sleep?
* Are there any problems in your relationship with your sexual partner?
* Does your partner have any sexual problems?
* Are you anxious, depressed or under stress?
* What medications do you take, including any herbal remedies or supplements?

- Do you drink alcohol? If so, how much?
- Do you use any illegal drugs?
- What, if anything, seems to improve your symptoms?
- What, if anything, seems to worsen your symptoms?

For a lot of blokes answering those questions honestly may tell the doctor all he needs to know to make a diagnosis and recommend a treatment.

If there's a concern that there's a deeper root problem (sorry) with your health then some tests might be needed. Some might seem a bit *personal*, but if you want to fix the problem (and be sure there's nothing life-threatening going on in the background) then grit your teeth and get 'em done!

Some of the possibilities are:

- *Physical exam.* This might include careful examination of your penis and testicles and checking your nerves for sensation.
- *Blood tests.* A sample of your blood might be sent to a lab to check for signs of heart disease, diabetes, low testosterone levels and other health conditions.
- *Urine tests.* Like what happens with blood tests, a sample of your pee is tested to look for signs of diabetes and other underlying health conditions.
- *Ultrasound.* Usually done by a specialist in an office, it involves holding a scanning device over the blood vessels that supply the penis. It uses sound waves to create a video image that lets your doctor see if you have blood flow problems. This test may sometimes be done together with an injection of medications into the penis to stimulate blood flow and produce an erection.
- *Overnight erection test.* Most men have erections while they sleep without remembering them. This simple test involves wrapping a special device around your penis before you go to bed. This device measures the number and strength of erections that are achieved overnight and can help to determine if your 'erectile dysfunction' is related to psychological or physical causes.
- *Psychological exam.* Either your doctor or a specialist might ask questions to screen for depression and other possible psychological causes of your problem.

The first thing your doctor should do after the test results are in is to make sure you're getting the right treatment for any health conditions that are found. That should happen whether or not they could be causing or worsening the sex problem that brought you to the doctor in the first place.

Next: treatment. That's going to depend on the causes and severity of the problem, and any other issues that the tests might have uncovered. Usually there'll be more than one option - your doctor can explain the risks and benefits of each treatment and should consider your preferences. Your partner's preferences also might play a role in your treatment choices, especially if you want to stay partners.

I'm not about to list every possible medicine or treatment you might have proposed to you, but here's a sample:

Oral medications. That's Viagra and stuff like it. Contrary to popular mythology, they're not aphrodisiacs and they don't give you an instant hard-on – someone still has to do some work on the old fella. What they *do* do is improve the blood flow to the muscles of the penis.

Possible side effects include hot flushes, a blocked nose, headache, affected vision, backache and stomach upset.

Talk to your doctor first – don't just buy stuff off the shelf or on-line. The drugs may not work or may even be dangerous if you:
- Take nitrate drugs — commonly prescribed for chest pain (angina)
- Have very low blood pressure or uncontrolled high blood pressure (hypertension)
- Have severe liver disease
- Have kidney disease that requires dialysis.

Herbal remedies. Pretty much everything I just said about oral medications also applies to the herbal 'alternatives'. If it hasn't been prescribed by a health professional who knows your medical history, I'd suggest you don't touch it.

The US Food and Drug Administration (FDA) has issued warnings about several types of "herbal viagra" because they contain potentially harmful drugs that are *not* listed on the label. The dosages might also be unknown, or they might have been contaminated during formulation. I'll go into a lot more detail about the pros and cons of supplements in Chapter 6.2.

Self-injection. With this method, you use a fine needle to inject a prescribed drug into the base or side of your penis. Each injection generally produces an erection that lasts about an hour. Because the needle used is very fine, pain from the injection site is usually minor.

Side effects can include bleeding from the injection, an inconveniently or uncomfortably prolonged erection (yes, there is such a thing and it's called 'priapism') and formation of fibrous tissue especially if you keep sticking the needle in the same spot.

A suppository in the urethra. Sometimes called Muse therapy (don't ask me why – I don't see anything amusing about it) it involves using a special applicator to insert a tiny drug-filled suppository inside your penis. The erection usually starts within ten minutes and lasts between thirty minutes and an hour.

Side effects can include pain, minor bleeding in the urethra and formation of fibrous tissue inside your penis if you use them a lot.

Penis pumps. A warning up front – the ones advertised in magazines and sex ads might not be safe or effective. It's your money and your old fella you're risking, but if that's your preferred treatment ask your doctor to recommend or prescribe a specific model. That way, you can be sure it suits your needs and that it's made by a reputable manufacturer.

How it works is that a hollow tube is placed over your penis, and then a hand-powered or battery-powered pump is used to suck out the air inside the tube. This creates a vacuum that pulls blood into your penis. Once you get an erection, you slip a tension ring around the base of your penis to hold in the blood and keep it firm. Then remove the vacuum device.

The erection typically lasts long enough for a couple to have sex. Remember to take the ring off after you're done!

There are a couple of side effects to mention. You might suffer some bruising of the penis, and ejaculation will be restricted by the band. Your penis might feel cold to the touch – either you or your partner might find that a bit weird (although some others might think it's a turn-on).

Penile implants. This treatment involves surgically placing either inflatable or semi-rigid rods into both sides of the penis. Inflatable devices allow you to control when and how long you have an erection. The semi-rigid rods keep your penis firm but bendable.

Penile implants are usually not recommended until other methods have been tried first, but they are popular among men who have tried and failed more conservative therapies. As with any surgery, there's a risk of complications, such as infection.

Blood vessel surgery. In rare instances, leaking or obstructed blood vessels can cause erectile dysfunction. That definitely needs a doctor's diagnosis! If it turns out that this _is_ the case, surgical repair might be needed. That could mean inserting a stent in the blood vessel to keep it open (like happens with some heart surgery) or a bypass procedure to take the blood flow around the blocked or leaky bit.

> **Simply put:** if you're having trouble with sex, talk to your doctor. Trying to improve things without understanding the cause of the problem or any other medical issues going on, you risk doing more damage than good.

6.2 Improving and supplementing your diet

I spent a fair bit of time in Chapter 5 talking about diet because I really believe diet is more about prevention than cure. I really want to stress to the blokes who _aren't_ already bothered by the symptoms of ageing that it's something better avoided than fixed.

But if you're one of us who are 'already there', then I'll also stress that it's never too late!

Doctors and dieticians will tell you what to cut out and what to add in. They won't all necessarily agree on the detail, but you can rely on a few basics: less junk food, sugar and alcohol, probably more vegetables, fruit and good quality protein.

It can be worth getting some tests done to see if you really do have specific food intolerances. Don't forget, some of them can be cumulative. Just because you've eaten a particular thing for years, doesn't mean you can continue to do so. I'd been scoffing tomato sauce and tomato paste since I was a kid before they started to be a problem. It took time and pain to work out that they *were* an issue for me, too, but having cut them out of my diet (not easy when you love pizza) I'm enjoying not walking with a couple of sticks!

Difficult as cutting stuff out of your diet can be, adding new stuff in can be just as challenging when you've got decades of practice at "I'm not eating that!!!" under your belt.

No matter how well they're prepared, I still can't develop a taste for a lot of green vegetables. Especially the leafy ones like spinach, cabbage, Brussels sprouts and lettuce. (Trivia time: the smell from overcooked cabbage and Brussels comes from an organic compound containing sulphur.) Other blokes don't like fish. I've met some who don't like red meat, including one of the genuinely toughest pro wrestlers in the business!

So take supplements to address the shortfalls. It also addresses the points I made in Chapter 5 about food not being as good as it used to be. Getting more calcium into your body, or Vitamin A, or iodine or potassium or whatever, may be just what you need to overcome your particular problem.

The making and selling of nutritional supplements has become a huge industry. So big and so lucrative that now some drug companies are getting involved. That's kind of ironic, because most medicine (with the exception of antibiotics) doesn't cure disease. It treats symptoms.

If you're serious about using supplements to improve your health, it's important you look really hard at what you're taking. Don't just look for the cheapest option, because not all supplements are created equal.

It's like buying a car. There are things that you look for in your ideal purchase. High performance. Reliability. The quality of the technology behind the car. Reputation. Prestige (who else is driving one of these?). And yes, price.

You won't get a Mercedes for the price of a Mazda (or if you did you should be *really* suspicious) but looking for value means looking for the best results on the features that matter to you for the price you're willing to pay. Not just buying the cheapest tin box on wheels you can find, then cursing two weeks later when it's fallen apart at the side of the road *just* when you were on your way to somewhere important.

That said, price isn't a guarantee of quality, either. Some 'prestige' cars are overpriced lemons. Some high-priced vitamins and supplements are really flashily-packaged 'filler' with not much benefit per capsule. You want bang for your buck!

Here are some things to look out for when you're considering supplements:

- Just how much of the 'active ingredient' is in each tablet/capsule/ dose? Compare a few brands to see if there's a difference in what's in each 'unit'.

- There are 47 nutrients and nutrient categories that medical science has identified as 'essential' – vitamins, anti-oxidants, trace elements and minerals, and several essential fatty acids. How many of those are included in the product? If you're buying 'multi-vitamins' they should really *be* 'multi'.

- What's the 'bioavailability' of the active ingredients? That means: how easily can your body absorb them? If there's 100mg of magnesium in a tablet, will you actually get 100mg of magnesium out of it or is it in a form that will pass through your digestive system without breaking down? Are you flushing most of your expensive vitamins down the toilet?

- What are they actually made from? Some vitamin tablets have been known to use calcium carbonate as a base (and main ingredient by volume) to attach their 'good stuff' to. That's chalk, mate, and I'm not keen on paying good money to eat chalk, no matter what's been stuck to it.

- 'All natural ingredients' needn't mean much either. Green tea leaves are a natural ingredient, but they may be carrying pesticides, fungicides or fertilizers that you *don't* want added to your body. Even without the chemical nasties, you have to ask how good is the source that the ingredient came from. Remember what I said earlier about the quality of a lot of the crops and vegetables now being sold?

- How good is the manufacturing process? Being 'laboratory made' doesn't tell you much. Toilet cleaner and metal polish can be made in a laboratory too. There's no law that says *they* have to be pharmaceutical grade. Funnily enough, there's no law like that for vitamins and supplements, either.

- Is there anything potentially dangerous in there? For instance, iron can become toxic if taken at high doses for a long period. Unless you're actually iron deficient you shouldn't be taking it – there should be enough in your normal diet – and yet there are multivitamins out there that are loaded with iron.

- How careful have they been in manufacture? Is their processing certified as pharmaceutical grade, food grade, or made in Mrs. McGinty's kitchen on the same bench where she cuts up the dog's scraps?

- To address some of the above questions, ask: have they been independently tested and certified, by someone who knows what they're talking about? I don't think there are a lot of athletes, sports stars or other celebrities out there who are actually trained and qualified biochemists or even nutritionists. There may be some, but not as many as there are those who are just paid to endorse a product because they're famous. Instead, look for something like "accredited by NSF International Dietary Supplement Verification Program" or "approved by the Australian Therapeutic Goods Authority."

So, as with buying food – start by reading the label!

I admit that's not always going to help. In New Zealand, the labeling laws for these products allow labels so vague that they're virtually useless. Even in Australia and the US, where the laws are tighter, the language and technical terms can put a lot of blokes off. What they tell you can be downright incomprehensible.

I've found one helpful solution. It's a book.

Back in the late 1990's the Canadian government decided to support the use of nutritional supplements in the same way that they supported the use of medicines. (Someone in the Department of Health actually spotted that prevention was better than cure!) In order to ensure their money was being spent effectively they commissioned a study of what was on the market.

Headed up by Lyle MacWilliam, a company called Nutrisearch did the evaluation. The reaction of the Canadian Government, and the interest of the general public, was so high that the report was published in book form in 1999. It's caught on.

The *Comparative Guide to Nutritional Supplements* is in its 5th Edition, published in Australia, Canada, New Zealand and the US, and translated into French, Spanish, Chinese and Korean.

For the 2014 edition MacWilliam and his team tested several hundred broad-spectrum nutritional products. 241 of them qualified as multiple vitamin/mineral supplements, from 90 different manufacturers. These were evaluated across eighteen criteria relating to the content, completeness, potency, and 'bioavailability' of their ingredients. Some rated highly, some drastically less so.

I'm not going to tell you who "won". It's not a race, although I suppose those 90 manufacturers are all competing for the same dollars. I will say, though, that the *Guide's* ratings do NOT reflect market share, or price. If you want to use supplements to improve your health, get a hold of the *Comparative Guide to Nutritional Supplements*, and make an informed choice about what's likely to work best for you.

Having bought your good quality supplements, there are a few tips to making the most of them.

First of all: taking them is always better than not taking them, but the general recommendation is to take supplements with food, and spread evenly throughout the day with meals. For multivitamins especially it's best to take them just after a meal as many vitamins and minerals shouldn't be taken on an empty stomach due to poor absorption and accompanying nausea.

As a general rule it's a good idea to take your supplements in the morning because it gives them the best chance to be absorbed into your system and kick starts the day with a good nutritional foundation.

If you're taking multiple 'hits' of something, then after your breakfast dose try to take the rest with other meals throughout the day. Preferably spread the dosage evenly throughout the day for optimal results.

However different vitamins are suited to different times. Some are better first thing or later during the day – check the directions on the packageing. Personal preference and experience of knowing what works for you and your lifestyle also plays a role. You might realise you get the most from a particular supplement after a workout because it replenishes your energy, or before bed because it helps you to sleep better.

Whatever 'timetable' you find works best for you, I reckon you should try to take your supplements at the same or similar time each day. Your body gets into a routine and this helps the absorption of vitamins into your system.

Nutritional supplements aren't a 'magic bullet'. Sometimes some blokes will see dramatic benefits quickly. It depends on what their condition and circumstances are.

Be patient and persist. You can't see what's happening inside your body – that doesn't mean it isn't happening.

Simply put: a good diet and good quality supplements aren't a quick fix. They're a medium- to long-term strategy to improve your overall health from the inside out.

6.3 Change your lifestyle – change your life

Sometimes it seems the hardest part of making changes in your life is time management. You're already busier than you'd like – how do you fit stuff like exercise in?

It's a matter of changing patterns and habits. Replacing old ones with some that will serve you better.

I read a really good interview with the great fast bowler Glenn McGrath about how he looked after himself since giving up cricket. After years of having disciplined diet and training supported by professionals from Cricket Australia, how did he go when left to look after himself?

> "I think simply staying healthy and active is becoming increasingly difficult. People are so busy and it can be really hard to find the time to look after yourself. I think it's very important that people take responsibility for their own health by trying to stay active. It's also important that people are familiar with their bodies and have regular check-ups to ensure they stay as healthy as possible... early detection of an illness is really important."

A habit is something that's become so strongly wired into your brain that you can do it without thinking. They're thoughts, emotions or behaviours wired so deep that they've become automated – your brain running on autopilot.

Habits all have 'triggers'. You see or hear or do a particular something, then without even thinking about it, you do another thing.

Maybe as soon as your feet touch the floor beside the bed in the morning you go for a leak, then you brush your teeth. As soon as you sit in the car you put your seatbelt on, before you do anything else. You have your first mouthful of cold beer after work and immediately feel like a smoke. When you buy a coffee at the canteen you always get a pie and a doughnut to go with it, whether you're actually hungry or not.

They're all habitual behaviours – some good, some not so good. If you want to improve your health then you can start by improving some of those rusted-on habits.

Old habits never really die – the trick is to replace them with better ones. To do that you first need to do two things: identify the bad habit, and identify its trigger.

Want to cut down smoking while you drink? Buy a packet of nuts with that first beer. Instead of reaching for a ciggie to stick in your mouth, consciously stop yourself and very deliberately grab a couple of peanuts or cashews instead. When you do, make a point of telling yourself, "Yeah, these are better for me."

Trying to lose weight? When you order your coffee (try it with less sugar!) actually think about whether you really are hungry. If you are, look at your options. Fancy an apple or an orange? Do you really need both the pie *and* the cake? You might not be giving up doughnuts forever and ever, but if your new habit is to *think* about how you feel before announcing what you want to eat then you're doing well. Engage the brain before putting your mouth into gear.

"Your habits can take you towards your goals, or away from them."
- Michelle Duffield
Champion Ironman Triathlete

You might want to take a few steps beyond improving your diet.

If you're a **smoker**, you might decide to cut down or even quit. One good thing about our bodies are that they fundamentally know how to heal themselves.

- Twelve hours after your last smoke the increased level of carbon monoxide in your blood will be back to normal.
- Within a week much of the nicotine will be out of your body, and your senses of smell and taste will improve.
- In a month your skin will probably be cleaner and clearer.

- Within ten weeks of quitting, the membranes inside your lungs have been cleaned. Maybe not healed, but cleaned, so any damage gets no worse.
- Three months after you quit, you'll be breathing easier - your lung function will have improved.
- A year after you give up, your risk of heart disease is halved.
- If you've smoked a pack per day, by the end of a year you'll have saved over $7000, so your wallet will feel better too.

Get some **exercise**. Don't go crazy – listen to your body. For the sake of your heart, the recommendation from the British Heart Foundation is that the exercise be regular (30 minutes, five times per week) and aerobic. That means getting your heart rate up and feeling slightly out of breath. See that word? *Slightly.* Not wheezing and changing colour.

It's good for your brain, too. Regular exercise has been shown to do all these things for your little grey cells:

- Promote blood flow
- Deliver nutrients for cell growth and maintenance
- Control inflammation
- Improve insulin sensitivity so control your blood sugar better
- Expand the size of your memory centre
- Boost levels of a protein called BDNF.

BDNF ('brain-derived neurotropic factor', if you really want to know) is the key element in protecting neurons and more importantly, in creating the new synapses and connections that keep the brain functioning well despite ageing.

Aerobic exercise that gets your heart pumping (e.g. walking, not stretching) is the absolute best way to generate more BDNF – even reversing some of the damage that you may already be feeling the effects of. For instance, you might find your memory improving!

Try stuff out and see what works for you. Walking, cycling or jogging if your joints and back are up to it. Dancing, if the music makes it easier to zone out of the aches and pains as your body gets used to something new.

Help coach the local kids footy or cricket team – do some practices with them, *don't* try to compete with them (no matter how good you were twenty years ago). That does something positive for your community as well as for you.

"Exercise can be a lot of fun. It's not necessarily about being the best or the fastest – it's simply about getting outdoors and having a go, joining a local team with some friends or incorporating exercise into family activities."

- Glenn McGrath

Australian international Hall of Fame cricketer

Swimming or even just doing some exercise in the pool can be a good solution if your hips or knees or back are a problem. The water takes some weight load off those joints. But don't get lazy on it – remember, the idea is to get your heart rate up, not just flollop around enjoying the coolness. And I really do know how tempting that can be!

Aqua-aerobics can be really helpful, especially if your joints and muscles are out of practice at bearing your weight while you move it around a bit actively. The water really is a big help.

Most aqua-aerobics classes have a VERY high percentage of women. That can be off-putting, especially if you're self-conscious about the shape your body is in. Not all of those classes are especially welcoming of blokes, I know. Whether you turn up with a wife or girlfriend, or worse, unattached, there will be some women in the pool who will at the very least spend a lot of the class giving you "What the hell are *you* doing here?" looks, even if they don't call you a pervert out loud.

But if you really enjoy exercising in the water you have a couple of options:

- Persist. Keep trying until you find a class where you *are* made welcome.

- Talk to a trainer or occupational therapist – someone who really knows their stuff – and ask them to give you a program of stuff you can do in a pool without being in a 'class'.

I talked about resistance training back in Chapter 5.4. I've got good news for older blokes who haven't spent much time in the gym. Research has shown that if you start doing resistance training exercises and work on increasing your rates and/or weights as steadily but quickly as you can improve the rate you absorb and use protein in as little as two weeks.

I've read a study that reckons the average bloke loses about 4% of muscle strength every year after he hits 40. That's muscle quality, not muscle mass. If you're aiming to slow down or even reverse that, your best program in the gym is not lots of reps, but slow ones. Gradually increase the weights before you look at increasing the number of reps, and don't ramp up the speed. You'll improve muscle quality better by lifting and lowering slowly and steadily. And you're less likely to damage yourself.

Remember to take it easy. Challenge yourself, sure, but do it in small steps. If you've been a couch potato for ten years, don't start with a two hour run, or bench-pressing your own bodyweight. Set targets and work up to them or you can do more harm than good.

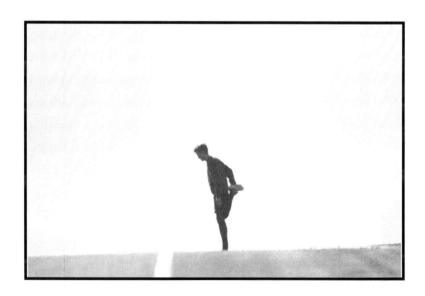

Don't underestimate the humble walk. The George Institute for Global Health reckons increasing your daily steps from 1000 to 10,000 can lower a sedentary person's chance of dying early by 46%. Even if you only increase by 3000 steps per day, five days per week, they reckon you'll delay death by 12%,

There was a study done in the UK in 2013 that examined the mental health benefits of walking outside in the country at least once per week. They weren't focusing on physical benefits – lots of studies have done that.

They found an 80% improvement rate in over 2000 subjects who started outdoor walking during the course of the study. These were people who'd been complaining of headaches, stress, anxiety – all the way up to diagnosed 'clinical depression'.

Getting out into 'the country' three times per week was suggested as optimum. That's not easy when you work in a big city, I know. But if you can find a park, or even a town square you can do a few laps of, they're a better option than a walking machine in a gym full of recycled 'air-conditioned' sweaty air.

Just being out in the fresh air is an obvious benefit. The study identified another big advantage of "non-urban" walking, especially for spells of over an hour at a time. It's the necessity of watching where you put your feet – you're 'in the moment' concentrating, so the brain can't keep focusing on whatever has been depressing you. A really healthy distraction!

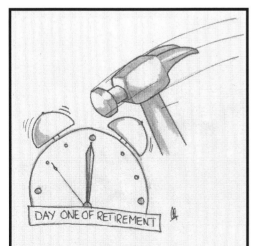

DAY ONE OF RETIREMENT

It might sound strange, but **retirement** can be a killer. I've known too many blokes who've passed away within a year of finishing work.

A couple have overdone their 'fresh start' and failed to survive the over-enthusiastic leap into lots of unfamiliar exercise.

But others have, I think, really died of boredom. After forty-odd years of having a regular routine they couldn't find new ways of spending the day.

Some sat at the bar from opening time until the money or the barman's patience ran out. That's tough on an ageing liver. Others just sat in a chair at home, staring at daytime television until they lost the will to live.

It wasn't that they ran out of money to live on. The problem was that their bodies, or their minds, pretty much wore out.

"There's a huge difference between well-being and being well off."
- Mitchell Kochonda
Gold Coast athletics preparation coach

If you haven't already got one, take up a **hobby**. If work is getting you down, or you feel you need to get away from the family more, then find something you enjoy doing.

It might be something competitive like golf or bowls or poker or bridge. Maybe a more solitary pursuit like fishing or cryptic crosswords. I know blokes who regard their 5-times-per-week gym visits as a hobby.

You might want to turn your hand and brain to something creative. Photography. Pottery. A good mate of mine took up painting-by-numbers just so he could learn a new skill. One of his first efforts hangs on my wall and I'm bloody proud to have it.

Is there a "Mens' Shed" anywhere near you? Try it out. That organisation, and others like it, are purpose-built for giving blokes something to do, and do it in company. You're not guaranteed to like everyone you meet there, which makes it very much like life really – but it beats loneliness and inactivity.

> ## "Some people live more in twenty years than others do in eighty. It's not the time that matters, it's the person."
> *- Doctor Who*
> Time Lord

I know an ex-builder who took up wood carving just to keep the smell of fresh-cut timber in his life. My hobby is cross-stitch. Okay, not the most macho choice in the world. My late wife introduced me to it years ago in the hope of teaching me patience and improving my temper – and it worked. It's like meditation for me (I'll talk more about meditation later). I get very focussed on the detail of what I'm stitching, and whatever else has been getting on my nerves just gets forgotten for a while.

That's the point: free your head from whatever is bringing you down. If what you choose actually generates a finished product that you can show off, use, sell, give away, or hang on the wall of your shed then so much the better!

Simply put: the way you live your life has a lot to do with the way you feel. If you want to feel better than you do now, you'll have to make some changes.

6.4 Look to the East

Eastern and Western medicine aren't mutually exclusive. Nor is it a matter of one being "right" and the other "wrong". Because of its focus on treating symptoms as quickly as possible Western medicine is especially good for 'emergency care' – dealing with sudden onset injuries and conditions that are a reaction to a specific incident (like poisons or allergies, or a heart attack from over-exertion). Eastern medicine is much more concerned with finding and treating the root causes of problems, and strengthening the body's own ability to defend against and cope with the sudden stuff.

I've heard it suggested that mid-life crisis is a uniquely 'Western' phenomenon. I don't buy that. Yu Yan ("call me Jack") is a friend in England who is a practitioner of what's called Traditional Chinese Medicine or TCM.

Jack is good. Very good. He's helped me with several problems, from a badly busted ankle to a persistent troublesome skin complaint. I asked him about the Chinese perspective on male mid-life crisis.

He described it as a "crisis of the spirit, triggered by all sorts of pressures." The Chinese expressions for it translate to 'the grey mid-life' and '40 year old man syndrome', although it often happens anywhere between 39 and 50.

The 'second phase of adulthood' between 40 and 60 should be the most fulfilling but it's also the most responsible. When you're young the world can forgive your being impulsive or silly (up to a point) but by middle age there's an expectation that you'll show your mature and responsible self. That includes recognising your own faults. A man may get to a point where he hates going to work, but he doesn't like being at home, either.

There is a long tradition, going back at least as far as the Yellow Emperor in the 2nd Century B.C., that when a man turns 40 it is the turning point of his health. Things go downhill from there, physically and mentally.

Jack listed six significant elements or events that may be part of a man's mid-life crisis – the time when "a man loses his smile":
1. Physical and mental decline, including greater susceptibility to illness
2. Greater sense of the heaviness of the burden of work and family responsibilities
3. Reduced confidence in both self and career prospects
4. Children assert their independence and leave home, changing the family structure
5. Responsibility for caring for elderly parents
6. Worry about the future and the impacts of age.

So, there's a fundamental difference with Western medicine for a start – where there is still resistance in a lot of quarters to the idea of male menopause even existing.

As to treatment, the differences are really striking.

There are five 'practices' within Traditional Chinese Medicine:

1. Acupuncture

2. Chinese herbology

3. Nutritional therapy ("food as medicine")

4. Exercise therapy (tai chi and qi gong - static and moving meditations plus breath exercises)

5. Manipulative therapy (massage, assisted yoga and tui na*)

(* Tui na is the sort of thing that chiropracters do – like bone and joint manipulation and soft tissue adjustment.)

A key to understanding Traditional Chinese Medicine is appreciating the idea that physical and emotional wellness are inextricably linked. Not just 'related' – what's going on with one has a direct impact on the other.

Twelve 'energy channels' or 'meridians' are identified, each relating to one specific organ and connecting to numerous other organs and points around the body. Energy, called 'qi' or 'chi' travels along and around those channels.

Those connections are key to things like reflexology and acupuncture: putting pressure on a spot on your foot, or a needle in the back of your hand, to treat a problem with your insides.

It's why an acupuncturist might stick a needle just below your knee to treat a problem with your spleen – it's not like he or she can reach inside and work directly on the organ, so the treatment is applied to a point from where the energy will go where it's needed.

Chinese medicine identifies a number of fundamental emotions. An excess of any of them, even the ones we think of as 'good ones', has an effect on the body, and it's a 'one to one' effect, each emotion playing on a particular specific organ.

Jack gave me five examples that I've worked into a table:

EMO-TION	AFFECTED ORGAN	EFFECT	SYMPTOMS
Happi-ness	Heart	Excess happi-ness can burn extra heart qi (energy)	Less concentration, diz-ziness, palpitation, poor sleep, at worst sudden collapse
Anger	Liver	Extreme an-ger can trigger over-excite-ment of liver qi, over-consump-tion of blood by the liver making it inefficient, once this anger heats the body it is difficult to cool down and rebalance so it can affect other organs.	Liver qi travels the wrong way, upsetting circulation and the digestive sys-tem. This can often cause bloating, abdominal pain or diarrhoea. At worst it can cause vomiting of blood, stroke, or even death.
Sadness/grief	Lung	Distress can cause lung qi blockage.	Tight chest, shortness of breath, difficulty breath-ing, gasping, coughing.

Anxiety/ worry/ brooding	Spleen	Excess concentration or over-thinking can block qi and blood flow in one place instead of flowing all over the body, thus causing illness.	Stomach & spleen out of order: digestion goes wrong, low appetite, bloating after eating, indigestion, constipation, diarrhoea. At worst, anaemia, water retention, lack of nutrition.
Fear	Kidney	Fear does not affect the kidney directly – it affects the heart after which the kidney takes the burden.	Damage to kidney essence and heart spirit, low spirits, sleepy, weak nervous system, low immune system, palpitation – worst case mental dysfunction.

Jack's advice is if you want to stay fit and healthy do not emotionally over react. Take a deep breath and stay in control of yourself.

If a body function is out of order for any other reason such as infection or injury, that in turn can cause all sorts of emotional symptoms. Furthermore, beyond the body/emotional interaction, other factors can also influence health – social factors like religion and community. That means the expectations that others have, or cause you to have of yourself.

So, to respond to all those factors Chinese medicine concentrates on healing the whole system, not just the symptom. That will usually mean applying not just one form of treatment but several. There is a focus on the target organ, organs and other parts of the body that are connected to it, and the energy pathways or channels ('meridians') that run between them.

I admit I was pretty cynical about the idea of these 'meridians' for a long time. Then one day in Singapore my feet were sore and tired and I wanted them massaged. The little old guy who was my masseur was also a reflexologist. As he worked away he pressed on one particular spot, and I jumped. I mean really jumped.

"Ah-hah," he said. "You have kidney problem."

"I had surgery for kidney stones a few weeks ago," I admitted.

He smiled and nodded, and kept working. A minute or two later, he hit a different spot. I didn't jump this time, but I squirmed in obvious discomfort.

"Liver not good," the old guy said with something like an evil grin.

Anyone who knows me and knows how fond of a drink I was for a very long time won't be surprised at his instant diagnosis. But the kicker for me came a few minutes later when the old bloke found yet another point on my foot that caught his attention.

He pushed and poked at it, obviously expecting me to react like I had for the other two spots.

"What wrong with your gall bladder?" he demanded.

"I don't have one. Surgeon took it out years ago."

He smiled and got on with the job, and I thought, 'There really is something to this reflexology stuff!'

It explains why one of the primary tools of a good TCM practitioner is what's called *pulse diagnosis*. The therapist will feel for twelve pulse points on your hands, one for each of the meridians. Some are superficial, some are deep. He or she will feel for subtle irregularities in the rhythm or strength of the pulse that indicate that a problem.

The actual problem itself might be at any point along the meridian, but the symptoms could show up anywhere (although the main organs are the most likely culprits).

So, with that thought of interconnectedness in mind, here are some examples from Jack Yu Yan of treatments that might be applied to four of the conditions mentioned above:

Excess happiness:
- acupuncture and acupressure on the pericardium and heart meridians – improving energy, evening blood flow, calming the mind. Some herbal medicine can help.

Anger:
- acupuncture and acupressure on liver and gall bladder channels – unblocking the qi energy, detoxing rubbish created by emotions, transporting blood and nutrition to where they should be. Goji berry, chrysanthemum and dark plum mix tea will help.

Rumination:
- acupuncture and acupressure on stomach channel, strengthening spleen and stomach function, improving the digestive system and its absorption function, keeping energy flow smooth. Again, some herbs will help, such as a blend called *shenling baizhu san*. I can't really offer a useful translation, sorry. It's a compound of several ingredients, some of which have names in Latin and Chinese but not in common English.

Fear:
- acupuncture and acupressure on all points of the kidney meridians – strengthening kidney essence, delaying body degeneration, improving memory and work efficiency, releasing pressure. The medicine *liuweidihuang wan* (another un-translatable compound!) should help.

The oldest therapeutic form of Chinese medicine is "qi gong" (pronounced "chee gung"). It's a form of the 'exercise therapy' that goes beyond the application of medicines and physical interventions like Jack explained. It aims to improve mental and physical health by integrating postures, movement, breathing and focussed meditation.

The idea is to help the body strengthen and heal itself, notably:

- Immune system
- Internal organs
- Nervous system
- Hormonal system
- Pain relief
- Stress and emotional release.

You might find reference to both 'health qigong' and 'medical qigong'. The difference, according to the website of the Australian Institute of Medical Qigong is:

> "Health qigong is a set of exercises that are performed to promote general health. Medical qigong involves the diagnosis and treatment of a particular individual's specific physical, mental, emotional and spiritual imbalances. As such, it can be used to treat specific medical conditions as well as a tailored means of maintaining general health and well being."

So if you're considering qi gong as a treatment, ask the question, "Are you offering a general solution or one that's specifically for *me*?"

Simply put: Traditional Chinese Medicine is all about addressing root causes, not symptoms, and treating the whole patient, not just the 'sick bits'.

You might also decide to investigate Reiki or Seichim. They both are healing therapies based on the manipulation of energy in and around the body.

A practitioner using either of these methods will channel healing energies that resonate with your bodies own energies – identifying and correcting imbalances.

Albert Einstein reckoned that energy and matter are fundamentally the same thing. If you accept that, then you can see a logic in how repairing energy can translate into repairing organs and flesh.

If you're interested in the option, talk to a practitioner. They may wave some qualification papers, but bear in mind that there isn't a Reiki equivalent of the AMA, a truly comprehensive industry body, or independently-regulated formal qualification. There isn't a recognised University course like the one that produces doctors and surgeons. That doesn't mean that the best of them don't know their discipline and aren't committed to healing.

A good therapist will tell you that the key to these therapies working (or not) is really the extent to which you believe in them yourself. The body's natural tendency is to heal itself – provided it's given a fighting chance to do so. Someone drawing symbols in the air above your middle isn't likely to be enough to cure your kidney complaint, no matter how strong your belief, if there aren't some other steps taken. Medicine. Lifestyle changes.

The other side of that coin is that if you've got yourself convinced that you'll "never get better" then no amount of treatment, of any sort, will make you feel well.

> **Simply put:** if you don't really believe a treatment will work, you're very probably going to prove yourself right.

6.5 Getting to the point - acupuncture, acupressure and 'bodywork'

Peter Lecke is a licenced acupuncturist with a lot of study and professional practice behind him. As a relatively young bloke he suffered from chronic severe knee pain but was reluctant to undergo the replacement surgery that was being offered as the 'best option' by his doctor. In desperation he went to an acupuncturist. One short program of treatment later his knees felt fine.

But what struck Peter even more (and prompted him to study, then practice Chinese medicine) was that after the acupuncture for his knees, he realised that he suddenly didn't have the digestion troubles that had plagued him for years – the bloating and cycle of diarrhea/ constipation were suddenly gone.

In Chapter 6.4 I talked about 'meridians' – energy channels that connect organs and other parts of the body.

Acupuncture and acupressure are all about working directly on those meridians. There are over 2000 'points' identified in the textbooks. Stimulating the nerves at the correct combination of points is the means of healing an enormous range of problems and conditions.

Acupuncture - a jab well done

Acupuncture is one of the oldest, most commonly used medical practices in the world. It is believed to have originated in China more than 2,500 years ago, gaining attention in the West in the 1970s, when China and the U.S. opened relations. The practice has been growing in popularity since, including within the 'conventional' medical profession. Many doctors are now choosing to train in acupuncture as another string to their therapeutic bow.

It's probably the most accepted and 'Westernised' element of traditional Chinese healing. According to the Johns Hopkins University School of Medicine & Hospital in Baltimore, Maryland:

> "Acupuncture theories today are based on extensive laboratory research and have become widely known and accepted. In addition, controlled studies have shown evidence of the effectiveness of acupuncture for certain conditions. At present in the United States, about 3,500 doctors and 11,000 to 12,000 nondoctor acupuncturists use this medical art. About 40 acupuncture schools train nondoctors and about 500 to 600 doctors, according to the American Academy of Medical Acupuncture."

The World Health Organisation has an on-going study clinically testing just how well acupuncture really works. So far they've listed over

300 conditions that it's been *proven* to effectively treat. There are about 600 more that they say 'evidence supports its effectiveness' in addressing.

> **"I am convinced that acupuncture is going to be one of the greatest contributions that any group of people has made to the future of all medicine, if it is handled correctly by the people of the Western world."**
>
> - *Dr. W. Kenneth Riland*
> Personal physician to President Richard Nixon

So how does it work? Traditionalists explain that acupuncture points (where the needles go) stimulate the flow of qi energy. The 'Western scientific' explanation is that they are stimulating the central nervous system. That releases chemicals into the muscles, spinal cord, and brain. These chemicals either alter the experience of pain or release other chemicals that influence the body's self-regulating systems.

Peter Lecke gave me five examples of how acupuncture works – effects clinically supported by the WHO studies:

- Augmenting of the immune system by raising the white blood cell count and levels of specific hormones

- Pain management by stimulating the secretion of endorphins

- Neurotransmission interference by affecting levels of serotonin and noradrenalin

- Increasing or decreasing blood circulation to an affected area by constricting or dilating blood vessels, e.g. by stimulating the release of histamines

- Closing certain nerve 'gates' by strategically overloading them with impulses, thus blocking pain transmission.

> **Simply put:** acupuncture works by activating your body's own healing and pain control systems.

Peter reckons that acupuncture treatments are most effective when done in a short timeframe. Three treatments in three days work better than one per week for three weeks. It allows the benefits to build on each other quickly.

I know that when Jack did three treatments in successive days, the ankle that I'd rolled and twisted went from the size and shape of a large grapefruit on Saturday morning (when I couldn't put any weight on it), to normal size and shape and being walked on by Monday afternoon. On previous occasions bandaging, ice, and anti-inflammatories had taken weeks to have a comparable impact.

Dr. Bill Meyers, the Federal President of the Australian Medical Acupuncture College (AMAC) is honest enough to admit to me that while most people have a positive response to acupuncture, up to 15% report no benefit. That might be something to do with the practitioner, or the patient, or even the condition itself. But it's still pretty good odds!

There are doctors, including G.P.s, out there who offer acupuncture as part of their general practice. They're worth looking out for. Especially if they're members of AMAC or its local equivalent. If you are in Australia there may even be a bit of Medicare rebate available (private health fund rebates don't apply to G.P. services, unfortunately).

I've read of one medical 'expert' who reckons he'd "rather stick his head in a bucket of water than have acupuncture". Based on my experience, that's his loss. But as with all these options, the only way to find out if it works for you is to try it. Just look for someone professional. It's a science, not 'folk medicine'.

E-STIM - wired for sound health

Transcutaneous Electronic Nerve Stimulation (TENS), or E-STIM has been endorsed and used by the Western medical profession for decades. You can now buy units to 'do-it-yourself' at home! When done correctly the same key points targeted by acupuncture are stimulated by electronic or electromagnetic impulse. A pair of wires does the work of a needle, directing current flow through the cells associated with the area requiring treatment, producing the same biochemical reactions.

The basic principles are the same. The nervous system or qi energy is stimulated to promote healing, anaesthesia or both. What differs is the directness of the 'delivery system'.

Acupuncture is (pardon the pun) straight to the point. A well-trained, capable practitioner can insert a needle at a precise spot. Electromagnetic stimulation, even when applied by a specialist, affects not just the point but also the tissues around it. That may or may not be desirable depending on the circumstances and condition being treated.

Without specialized training the question of exactly where to apply the stimulus, whether by needle or by electrical impulse, is largely guesswork. This guesswork is made more complicated by considerations like referred pain disguising the true source of the problem, and the potential to do more harm than good by inappropriate treatment of the wrong (or even the right) spot.

Perhaps it's a psychological thing – a natural wariness of sharp objects – that has prevented "do-it-yourself at-home acupuncture" from making a big impression in the marketplace. Yet the electronic equivalent is selling well.

If you intend to treat yourself, get good professional guidance first. Have the problem properly identified, and find out <u>exactly</u> where the terminals of your nerve stimulation unit should be applied.

Done by hand - acupressure & bodywork

Those meridians and pressure points can also be manipulated other than by needles and electrical currents. They can just be pressed or kneaded by hand. That's acupressure, or 'bodywork'. I like that last term – it reminds me of a panel beater taking the dents out of a car. When the car body is straight it handles and performs better. Take the kinks out of your body and it should do the same.

Warren Hirst is a mate of mine who began his career with bodywork back in 2004. He's studied Acupuncture, Remedial Massage, Shiatsu, Swedish Massage, Dry Needling and has a Bachelor of Clinical Science degree. Having completed these courses in Thailand, South Africa, England and Australia, Warren brings a wealth of international knowledge and experience to the conversation.

When I talked to him about his perspective on male menopause he said:

"Every man is unique, has different DNA, lives in different circumstances, has different support structures and comes from a different background. So what may affect one person may have barely any effect on another. Many factors come into play when determining how men deal with their lives in their forties."

The blokes that Warren sees are typically coming to him first and foremost as a "massage therapist". They're troubled by all sorts of stiffness and soreness, and limited range of movement.

By using the right mix of acupuncture, shiatsu and remedial massage Warren eases up the cramped and tight muscles, releases and relaxes tendons and ligaments (that are often the real cause of what we think is 'joint' pain).

The blood flow is stimulated so there's more oxygen being delivered around the body. His work also unblocks that qi energy I mentioned earlier so it also flows around the body more freely. That combination boosts the person's overall vitality - i.e. just makes them feel better!

One temporary downside is that bodywork also shifts toxins that have built up in the painful area. That can lead to headaches or even a bit of nausea. It's why masseurs and other physical therapists will tell you to drink plenty of water after a treatment. It's not because you'll be thirsty, it's to allow your body to flush out the toxins that have been released into your system. Otherwise they'll probably just pool somewhere else, like in your brain (there's the headache) or kidneys if there isn't enough water pushing them through.

Once those toxins are out of your system though, you should feel a lot better. The physical improvement also often translates over into feeling better psychologically and emotionally.

Warren tries to promote that further during a consultation by looking into the lifestyle, how that relates to the symptoms and what the person could do to eradicate or lessen the symptoms.

> "I see myself as assisting people for 1 or maybe 2 hours a week. The other 166 hours are up to them. When they leave the clinic, they leave with a sense of wellbeing or the 'feel good factor'. They are taking care of themselves, and that leaves them feeling positive. Hopefully, this can spill over into other hours and days of the week."

Simply put: Acupuncture and bodywork may not be the solution to major trauma or a life-threatening disease, but they can be powerful weapons to help your body fight those things itself.

6.6 Homeopathy - using a little to tackle a lot

I was talking to a bloke I see in the pub sometimes about homeopathic remedies. His first joking response was, "No mate, I'm straight." But he then asked me, "Isn't it like that Chinese stuff?"

Only very faintly. Homeopathy is actually an old Western tradition: founded in what is now Germany in the late 1700s, and since then practiced widely throughout Europe.

Its resemblance to Chinese medicine is in the use of natural products as medicine, and in the fundamental belief that the body has the ability to heal itself. But where the two philosophies go from that starting point is quite different.

Homeopathy is based on the idea that "like cures like." The thinking is, if a substance would cause a symptom in a healthy person, giving the person a very small amount of the same substance may cure or prevent the illness. A dose of homeopathic medicine is meant to enhance the body's normal healing and self-regulatory processes.

A homeopathic health practitioner will use pills or liquid mixtures containing only a little of an active ingredient (usually a plant or mineral) for the treatment of disease. These are highly diluted products – you might hear them called "potentiated" substances.

There's a lot of debate around this particular treatment option, but there is some evidence to show that homeopathic medicines may have helpful effects. I have to say, though, there are some diseases and conditions that homeopathic treatment does _not_ work for. Cancer. Heart disease. Major infections or allergic reactions.

It's also important to talk to your medical doctor if you decide to use homeopathic remedies. There are some drugs that can lose their effectiveness, and others that can make a toxic cocktail when combined with the wrong thing.

So, given how homeopathy works, is it effective in dealing with male menopause? Strictly speaking, no, because what homeopathy does is promote the body's own natural function, and progressive changes to your hormone levels are part of that functioning.

However, as I've said before, there's often a lot more going on at 'middle-age' than just the decline of testosterone. The cumulative effect of a lot of stuff can be starting to kick in, both physically and psychologically. Homeopathy can potentially have a role in managing those effects.

Some of that is because as part of their 'whole of body' approach, homeopaths tend to pay particular attention to a patient's state of mind. That doesn't always sit comfortably with blokes.

Karen Phillips is a Canadian homeopath. She made this observation:
> "I usually see a lot more female than male, because I think men usually don't take care of themselves- they neglect their health and they don't like to talk. I think 75% of my practice are female, regardless of what disease they have. And, those men that come it's because their wife has forced them to come. Also, because alternative medicine is a lot more accepted by women than by men. Men are very engineer minded, very mechanical in their approaches - they have a very hard time to believe that something that conventional medicine has not put their seal of approval is of any value. Women are not like that. I think women are a lot more open to explore and investigate."

If you'd like to challenge Karen Phillips' assertion and do some exploration of what homeopathy might do for you, then go right ahead.

Brian Kaplan has practised as a homeopathic doctor for over 20 years. He reckons that over his career he's heard hundreds of 'mid-life crisis' stories. In most cases they weren't the reason the patient first came to see him. The man may have come in for just about anything. But in homeopathy, in contrast to orthodox medicine, the doctor must ask the patient not only about his illness, but about his whole life. That means talking about job satisfaction, his marriage, relationships with his children, hobbies and hopes and dreams. Brian reckons general practitioners are often too busy to ask about anything except the presenting problem.

As far as the actual remedies are concerned, what's prescribed will depend on what symptoms are presented, and what issues are recognised as being behind them. The remedy is intended to reflect the physical symptoms of the deeper issue. By getting the body to come to terms with the symptoms, the issues themselves become resolved. Here's a sample of remedies and their uses that Brian has suggested.

Lycopodium: useful for men who have a problem with commitment anyway, and now that life is going through a hard phase, have started to wonder if they married the right person in the first place. Otherwise (or also) they may be starting to experience some symptoms of sexual dysfunction.

The same remedy is also useful for a bloke suffering from what might be described as "Fear of being unable to reach his destination." As life reaches its mid-point, it starts to dawn on some men that they may never realise the dreams of their youth. Time is simply running out and this fills them with dread. Brian does admit, though, that it's possible however that men who always needed Lycopodium as a constitutional remedy have a higher incidence of or tendency towards this particular fear.

Natrum muriaticum: a remedy used for 'silent grief'. The bloke who keeps everything bottled up inside. He has an aversion to sympathy and will seldom seek counselling or advice of his own accord.

Aurum metallicum: for deep depression. It may be someone who's thinking or talking of suicide. But it also commonly suits successful, powerful men who distract themselves from their grief or depression, or avoid facing the challenges of middle age by "throwing themselves into their work" and becoming workaholics. These men tend to be successful and can even be very wealthy. They may look quite contented to colleagues and friends but inside they feel deeply depressed. They may even entertain suicidal thoughts which, when acted on come as a complete surprise to everyone around them.

Staphisagria: used in cases of repressed anger, resentment, sudden outbursts of bad temper, high and/or aggressive sex drive. Useful in instances when there is resentment at not being promoted or a man's not doing the work he hoped to be doing by the time he reached the age he's at.

Phosphoric acid: for the guy who isn't so much depressed as apathetic, listless, or indifferent to what's going on in his life. He has little enthusiasm for anything.

"The mass of men lead lives of quiet desperation."

- Henry David Thoreau

American writer and philosopher 1817-1862

Clearly, there's no "best remedy" for male mid-life crisis. The list above touches on only a handful of the things blokes may suffer from.

Brian Kaplan reckons that in his experience there are five main areas of concern that often seem to come up: sense of mortality, unsatisfactory or failing marriage, and disillusionment with family, work and/or the leisure pursuits that used to be enjoyed.

Unlike orthodox medicine, homeopathy really encourages people to talk about their whole lives. Just speaking to an empathic listener about what the trials and troubles feel like can be of great therapeutic benefit. Many men may turn up their noses at counselling and psychotherapy but may be prepared to reveal a lot to a doctor who is prepared to listen. Homeopaths tend to consider themselves "listening doctors" so the consultation process itself can be very helpful. Plus, the right homeopathic remedy may be just the tonic!

Simply put: there are two elements of homeopathy that could help – the 'whole of body' approach that considers what's going on behind the symptoms, and the remedies that may deal with the symptoms themselves.

6.7 Massage - there's the rub!

You might reasonably ask, "What does massage have to do with male menopause or midlife crisis?" After all, massage is just about a bit of self-indulgence, or maybe some treatment after sports or heavy work, right? Wrong.

According to a masseuse I met in Sydney, by alleviating stiffness and pain, it can make you feel better! But more than that, by improving muscle tone and circulation, Thai massage can slow down ageing.

That made some sense to me. When your circulation is working well then you're flushing out toxins (so they don't pool in kidneys or heart or anywhere else and do lasting damage), and moving energy around so that all of your cells have a chance of working well. That's why a well-trained massage practitioner will tell you that massages aren't technically supposed to "relieve stress", but instead act as a healing method for ailments (physical tension being one of the ailments).

The benefits aren't limited to Thai massage. There are several different types that differ in terms of their theoretical bases, techniques and oils used – which you choose to go for will depend on your needs and preferences.

Swedish Massage

What we now call "Swedish massage" is a classic Western massage (whether or not it is really Swedish is a subject of debate) whose techniques are based on the 'conventional' elements of anatomy and physiology. It's based on the same principles as modern Western medicine – treat the area where the problem (pain, tightness) is evident. The massage therapist targets your problem and massages the area. Simple.

That means it's focused on working directly on muscles and joints, as opposed to "energy flows" or "meridian points". Swedish massage is relaxing, often employing long strokes, kneading and tapping.

The Swedish massage is probably the most relaxing. It uses five different strokes to improve health. These strokes are sliding, kneading, rhythmic tapping, cross fibre, and vibrating. Swedish massages can improve wellness by:

- Reducing joint stiffness
- Reducing pain
- Improving osteoarthritis patients' movement range and functionality.

Traditionally you should be nude for a Swedish massage, but the term "massage parlour" has become so commonly used for brothels that a lot of the genuine therapists are now shying away from asking clients to strip off completely. If you *do* visit a genuine therapeutic massage house and they ask you to strip down to the buff, *please* don't then try to crack on to the person giving the massage.

Another prominent feature of Swedish massage is the use of oil. Types of oil include jojoba, shea butter, and other oils you find in skincare stores, or produced by big corporations.

A lot of therapists choose their oil based on principles of aromatherapy, adding essential oil/s to one of the neutral bases. So if you have an allergy or aversion to a particular oil or fragrance (e,g, I love cinnamon in food but the oil burns my skin like too long in the sun, while a mate of mine sneezes uncontrollably near lavender) let them know before they mix the essential oil into the base.

One variation on this 'Western' style that you may find is "deep tissue massage", sometimes called medical massage. This applies deep pressure to release chronic muscle tension. The massage therapist targets the farthest down muscle tissues, tendons and fascia (that's the protecting layer around muscles, bones and joints). By going so deep, it realigns the deeper layers of muscles and connective tissue.

While it can feel quite uncomfortable at the time, this can be very beneficial for chronic aches, tightness, soreness and pains.

Thai Massage

In its home country Thai massage is mostly used as a form of medicine, and can be painful for the uninitiated.

The massage therapist might start by placing you on a mat in various yoga-like positions for an hour or two, although this is less common the further you get from South-East Asia.

Thai massage uses deep and prolonged pressures that are done rhythmically by the therapist who leans a lot of their weight onto your body.

There is plenty of pushing and pulling in the Thai massage, and you'll often find your body in awkward positions. I remember one in particular that felt like I was on the wrong end of a really tough 30 minute pro wrestling match.

So Thai massages aren't in themselves stress-relieving, but your body will feel extremely, extremely supple and relaxed once the massage is over. Thai masseurs also frequently use their elbows to apply really intense pressure to specific points, which isn't common in the Swedish massage.

Massage oils are not a prerequisite in Thai massage, but you will most likely be given the option to have oils used. The oils are often traditional Thai concoctions that include lime, lemongrass or ginger.

Traditional Chinese Massage

Usually performed by Traditional Chinese Medicine practitioners, you won't often find genuine therapeutic Chinese massage at regular massage parlors or spas. Highly technical, this form of massage requires in-depth knowledge of the principles of Chinese medicine, i.e., meridian lines, energy flows and the like.

Traditional Chinese Massage is a very broad category, and methods used will depend on the practitioner and on your needs. Broadly though, they all focus on applying pressure at various points along the body's meridians (energy channels) to improve health.

Reflexology applies this principle specifically to 'meridian points' on the feet (or sometimes hands or even ears).

The masseur will focus on applying physical pressure to the same meridian lines or points that an acupuncturist would target. They will use their hands or sometimes a handheld device to do this.

One common technique is the "one finger technique", which addresses specific acupressure points on your body. The point of it is often to strengthen internal organs, heal injuries or get your *qi* flowing properly again, which may make it a particularly useful type of massage for a bloke feeling the drama of the years to investigate.

Massage oils as we commonly understand them are not used in Traditional Chinese massages, although some concoctions may be applied on you based on your condition. You may be given herbal medicine afterwards, as well.

Be warned: like the Thai version, Chinese massages can be quite painful because they aim to apply pressure to very specific points. Don't be afraid to tell your massage therapist that it hurts!

Perhaps more than any of the other Eastern massage types, Chinese is intended to address both overall health *and* specific medical conditions. For instance, some quite particular health benefits that are credited to Chinese massage include:

- Reducing nausea
- Alleviating pain
- Calming headaches

Traditional Indian Massage (Ayurvedic)

Like Chinese medicine, Indian medicine is a huge, huge branch of study, incorporating Ayurveda and other systems of medicine as well, like Traditional Tamil Medicine, which is a separate thing altogether.

Unlike other forms of massage, Ayurvedic massages often use poultices – or bags filled with ingredients like rice, herbs and fragrant oils. These poultices are pressed directly onto your body.

Other types of Indian massage are more conventional, and often use oils derived from traditional regional plants.

Japanese Shiatsu

Shiatsu is very similar to Chinese massage, for the simple reason that that's what it was based on when it emerged in Japan in the early 20th Century (becoming well-documented and 'organised' in the 1940's).

The key difference is that Chinese massage, like Chinese medicine, is more focused on 'total' wellness than Shiatsu, which focuses on a particular problem area.

Both recognise the interconnectedness of meridian points and the importance of energy flow. Broadly though, the Chinese approach is to heal the whole, and the afflicted area will be repaired as part of that process – whereas the Japanese approach is to use the relevant parts of the whole to target the problem.

By 'problem' I don't just mean an area of physical pain like a damaged joint – Shiatsu is also used to treat issues like depression, headaches, tiredness and digestive problems.

Again, you should be aware that because it involves applying pressure – sometimes strong pressure – on particular points, Shiatsu can be uncomfortable, even painful, when you first experience it.

If you are finding a massage – any type of massage – acutely painful, tell the masseur or masseuse to back off a bit. They may tell you that "it's meant to hurt" and to some extent that may be true, but pain is also your body's way of telling you something is wrong. Don't let your macho pride ("Can't... urgh... admit that... it hurts... ow... she'll think I'm... aargh... a wimp...") cause you bigger problems.

'No pain = no gain' is fine in theory, but a good therapist should know when to ease off. But he/she needs you to tell them when a line is being crossed. The risk of doing damage (or further damage) is quite real and pain is an important indicator of that possibility.

Remember – you're paying for the service – you have the right to say, "Hold it – that bloody hurts!"

Simply put: at the very least a good massage will relax you. At its best it can help heal some chronic problems.

6.8 Medical meditation – thinking yourself healthier

For a lot of blokes the word 'meditation' conjures up images of a bunch of hippies sitting in a circle watching a candle and humming to themselves.

It's actually a lot more complex than that, and there are a lot of ways to approach meditation. I've found the best of them (when you tackle them the right way) to be very, very good for your peace of mind. There is a school of thought that it can do, and be, considerably more.

An Oxford University study found that meditation helped 70% of participants get off depression medication. It's called 'mindfulness' – getting your head totally into the thing you're doing so that you stop thinking about whatever is stressing you.

It could be almost anything. A colouring book. Woodworking. Fly fishing. Sitting on a rock watching the waves roll in. The point is to focus on it so completely that you forget about work, family, the crap on the nightly news, all of it.

If you try it and find it's doing some good for your state of mind, then you won't be surprised to hear that there are those who say meditation can be as good for the body as for the mind.

Dr. Dharma Singh Khalsa is a rare type of individual – both physician (a certified specialist in anesthesiology, pain management and anti-ageing medicine) and a practising yogi.

His particular discipline is something called *kundalini* yoga. In the simplest terms I can muster, that's about absorbing healing energy into the body, and distributing it to where it's needed.

Dr. Khalsa and Cameron Stauth have written a book called *Meditation As Medicine*. It has some ideas and suggestions you might find useful.

Their take on meditation is that it's not just about 'relaxing and feeling better' – it's a lot more targeted than that. Khalsa and Stauth reckon, "No illness exists on just the physical, or just the psychological, or just the spiritual level." So they reckon that looking after your health means taking care of the spirit, the mind *and* the body.

Their approach is to nurture what they call the ethereal energy system, which transfers this nurturance to the physical body.

The means of transfer is via the eight chakras. These are defined as 'seven whirling vortexes of ethereal energy that are vertically aligned along the spine and head, plus the aura of ethereal energy that surrounds the entire body." The seven physical chakras are located in the same area as both a major nerve plexus and an important endocrine gland.

Simply put: 'chakras' are centres of physical or other energy that align with key points in the body's nervous system.

The second chakra is the one most relevant to the male menopause symptoms already mentioned. It's located behind the lower abdomen at the rear of the pelvis. Its nerve and endocrine structures are the sacral plexus and the Leydig cells respectively. The Leydig cells produce testosterone.

Medical meditation as Khalsa and Strauth present it aims to impact four major factors in impotence and libidinal dysfunction:

- vascular impairment,

- nervous system insufficiency,

- psychological problems,

- hormonal imbalances.

The program they propose, which by the way includes yoga (see Chapter 6.9) offers a range of benefits:

- restores blood flow,

- stimulates nervous system function,

- balances hormones (via the hypothalamic–pituitary axis),

- helps to discharge psychological stressors.

They suggest their techniques might also help blokes to overcome some of the most bloody aggravating symptoms of male menopause (age-associated hormonal decline they call it), including depression, lethargy, insomnia, and reduced libido. Like any shrewd therapy, Medical Meditation is touted as working best if it's combined with a sensible lifestyle program with the right combination of exercise, improved diet with adequate protein, hormonal replacement therapy if it's been recommended, appropriate herbal remedies, and food supplementation (see Chapter 6.2 above).

Khalsa and Stauth's book offers meditations that are specifically designed to "bring your second chakra to its highest state of function, and help you to solve real-world problems associated with energy imbalance in the second chakra." I'm not going to go into detail about the postures and mantras etc, but the book is very thorough. If you're struggling physically and you reckon that meditation might work for you then it's a good resource. Maybe not a 'starting place' though, if it's all completely new to you.

There are plenty of options available if you want to investigate meditation as a healing technique. If you don't want to jump in the deep end with the book *Meditation as Medicine* then dip your toe in the water with a session somewhere local. Maybe buy a 'guided meditation' CD or borrow one from the library. (Don't play it while driving please!) It can be very useful in dealing with psychological issues and depression, and sometimes those are at the true heart of physical symptoms.

Just be aware that meditation can also have side effects. A leading "alternative" health practitioner explained to me that, like medications, different *meditations* should be 'prescribed' to different people. Some conditions such as Bipolar Disorder and Schizophrenia risk being worsened with the wrong meditation for that condition. (I wish some doctors had been as aware, and as careful, with *medications* over the years!) However she reckons that for mild anxiety and depression, gentle 'mindfulness' meditation is proven to work.

> **Simply put:** meditation can be an effective way to clear the mind, and that can help heal problems with the body, too.

6.9 Yoga – mind bending as well as body bending

I read about a bloke named Andre Borschberg, a Swiss pilot & engineer who clearly enjoys a challenge. He spent 4 days, 21 hours and 51 minutes solo flying 8172 kilometres from Japan to Hawaii in a solar powered plane.

No easy task. The temperature got up to 37 degrees C in the cockpit. Across that time, two hours and nine minutes short of five days, he was resting only in intervals of twenty minutes. He was 62 years old.

I don't suggest that this is the sort of challenge you set yourself unless you've got a lot of relevant experience, but I was interested to know how he managed it. Andre reckoned the 'secret' was yoga. He credited yoga with being a "huge support" for sustaining a positive mindset and helping him to keep alert.

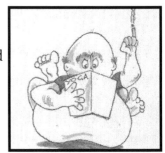

The point of that story is that yoga is about a lot more than sitting in strange postures and putting your back out.

I mentioned 'mindfulness' a little while back. Yoga is a very particular way of achieving the focus that takes you away from stress and pressure. Concentrating on a yoga posture means being very much 'in the moment'.

Celia Roberts BSc is the co-founder of the Yoga and Integrative Medicine Institute, an advocate for holistic health, with expertise spanning over 15 years.

She sees men suffering from back pain, shoulder pain, knee pain, and other signs of the body deteriorating, which is often why they've turned to yoga. Weight gain, addictions and headaches are also common, she told me.

As well as those struggling physically, Celia also often sees men with emotional or psychological issues.

Some feel that life has not lived to their expectations, and they report feeling depressed, lonely, or unhappy with their work or relationships. Blokes battling anxiety and high stress turn up at her practice as well.

She admits that one problem she faces is that "men are often less inclined to talk about how they are feeling, as opposed to female clients." So guys, if you're going to go talk to a specialist therapist (and this applies to any specialist in any field), be honest and open with them. They can't go into battle on your behalf without properly knowing what they're up against – that's not a fair fight!

Celia's belief is that we have to keep moving. Human bodies were designed to cover long distances on foot, not sit at a desk or behind a wheel all day. She recommends low impact activities – of which yoga is a prime example – as ways of extending both life expectancy and its quality.

Being outdoors, whether in a class or exercising on your own, is especially recommended for mental health. To that I'd add the rider: provided the air is reasonably clean in your outdoor area! See Chapter 5.6 for my thoughts on the air that we breathe.

It's worth noting Celia's observation that weight-bearing yoga exercises, done regularly over time, may even help to decrease the rate at which testosterone levels decline.

Don't expect immediate dramatic improvement. Take it steady and persist, allowing your strength and range of movement to build up gradually, especially if you know you're starting from a point of being really unfit. Celia says:

> "Quick and extreme fixes are not sustainable and often do more harm than good to the body and mind. Quick fixes may also hurt one's long term resolve if their goals are too extreme and unsustainable. I have had the great privilege of seeing

many male clients lose weight slowly over time and keep it off through steady and easy moderation of diet and exercise. Being able to keep their resolve way beyond their initial intent to lose weight is amazing to see, to further the resolve to eventually improve all areas of their life. This is the ultimate path of yoga; to move incrementally in small stages towards your goal."

Yoga has its risks, of course. Some postures might slow down recovery from an injury, or even cause more damage. That's why it's important that before you start a yoga program you spend time talking to the therapist about your health, and especially any physical limitations or problems you know you've got.

To have someone provide expert and individualised advice in the field of yoga therapy is a superior form of treatment, rather than starting out by just showing up to a general yoga class or buying a cheap Yoga DVD from the clearance bin. A good teacher will ensure you've got a good understanding of what you can and can't do. Then you can look at joining a group or exercising solo, knowing what you really want to achieve and how to achieve it safely.

> **Simply put:** yoga may help strengthen and even heal the body. It can also calm the mind and help you to both concentrate and relax.

6.10 Martial arts – fighting fit

If you reckon yoga isn't quite blokey enough for you, then maybe martial arts training is more your style.

It's not about hitting people and learning the best ways to hurt them. Yes, there's a strong element of learning to defend yourself, but that's not where the real benefits are, especially when it comes to your health.

True martial arts training is about self-knowledge, self-confidence and self-discipline.

Mr. Cooper Ali-Shabazz is a multi-medal winning martial artist. He's a teacher, philosopher, and author of a series of books on 'the Warrior's Way'. He's very clear about his concerns for blokes' health as they age.

> "The shame of the older man is that as he becomes older, after forty years, he lets himself go; he doesn't exercise, has become overweight and is physically weak. He may provide well for his family, and he works hard for this. But due to such hard work he neglects his physical well-being and fitness."

Shabazz recognises that some blokes are drawn to martial arts as an outlet for aggression, which is why, when he teaches, he puts so much emphasis on qualities like intelligence, righteousness and mercy. They're the sorts of things that distinguish a warrior from a thug. If you're considering a dojo or a teacher that doesn't clearly express values like that up front then you're not going to get the health benefits from the training.

The point is not to be an initiator of violence, but to learn how to react and respond. It's better to have that knowledge and never need it, than to one day need it and not have it. Underpinning real martial training is learning to overcome your own personal weaknesses, as well as the physical, emotional and psychological aggression of others.

Johnny Pink is another martial arts teacher. In his book *The True Value of Martial Arts* he writes:
> "Martial arts practice develops focus and creates positive changes within a person, which translates into better efficiency and a greater co-operation in the workplace environment."

Creating that positive attitude is the core of the real benefit of martial arts training for the older guy. Learning self-discipline in a structured way enables him to make changes that he'd previously struggled with – changes of diet or behaviour, for instance. Just taking action strengthens confidence.

The repetitious drills have physical benefits – they develop muscle tone, burn calories and increase cardio-vascular fitness. But they also have a psychological benefit. As the exercises become easier with repetition (as strength and flexibility gradually increase) that cultivates an attitude that says, "Yeah! I can do this!" They're also really good for 'letting off steam' – venting stresses and emotional pressures that otherwise build up and get suppressed.

I tense my right arm, draw my hand back to my opposite shoulder, and chop the side of my hand out into empty air, with as much force as I can. Four or five times, then do the same with my left arm. It's like the tension goes flying out of my hand. The knots in my shoulders and neck loosen up, and whatever has been bugging me seems less overwhelming. I don't need to be trying to break bricks or boards, but if that helps you to focus, fine. Work up to it though, please! If they broke easily we wouldn't make buildings out of them. Don't bust your hand – that'll only increase your stress.

I know that fitness programs and exercise classes can offer some of the same benefits. The difference that a good martial arts program offers is the context the physical activity is put into. Part of that is being taught to understand what Johnny Pink calls "universal principles that govern all human movement".

The other part is the encouragement of self-awareness. Not only becoming fitter, healthier, stronger, whatever – but recognizing and acknowledging it. I'll close this piece with Shabazz' thoughts on persistence and the power of the mind:

> "Start to see yourself differently and know that it is possible for you to change – to become who you want to be. If you are weak, become strong. If doubtful, then become decisive. Even if you don't view yourself this way today, start *thinking* differently and in time you *will* see change.
> Time is important. You cannot expect twenty to thirty years of unfocussed undisciplined thought to change overnight. It requires effort and time to strengthen the muscles of the imagination, mind and thought behaviour. But do not let anyone's negative opinion, nor the demons of doubt and mental weakness, deter you."

> **Simply put:** Martial arts training can offer the physical benefits of a good exercise program, as well as relieving stress and building self-confidence.

6.11 Articles of faith

Mid-life is a time of change for many blokes. For some, that includes turning to, or away from, religion.

I'm not going to tell you what to believe, or what not to. I've got my own faith and I reckon you're entitled to yours, whatever it is. But as far as health and healing is concerned, that word "faith" has a lot of power.

> **"Men are nearly always willing to believe what they wish."**
> - *Julius Caesar*
> 100 – 44 B.C.

One side of the coin is represented by things like the old witch doctor 'pointing the bone' at a believer, who is so terrified of what that means they give up on living – get sick and die. The other side is faith healing, when just the 'laying on of hands' makes someone suddenly feel well because they *believe* they are. (Maybe they were really a lot healthier than they thought, but had gotten so used to sickness it had become a habit. Whatever the reason, it certainly seems to work for some people.)

I don't reckon that sitting in a chair saying, "I *believe* I'm going to get better" without actually doing anything practical to help yourself has much chance of success. But I *do* believe that any therapy or treatment, conventional or 'alternative', has got NO chance of working for you if you go into it believing that it won't work.

"I'll try it, but it's never gonna work." Talk about self-fulfilling prophecy.

The stronger your belief that something is going to help you, the more chance there is you'll be right. Somewhere deep inside the brain, or the cells, the chemicals and reactions that enable the body to effectively heal itself get a kick along. And that can support the drugs, or exercises, or whatever else you're using to heal. Faith healing is not the same as having faith *in* your healing.

Organised religion doesn't work for me, although I've tried being deeply involved in it for a while. Some of the things that have been done in the name of one or other Church or creed over the millennia would surely make any self-respecting deity turn away and look elsewhere.

But being able to have a conversation in your head with God, Allah, a Creator, the Universe – whatever shape and name you choose – can be deeply comforting and even empowering. Call it prayer, call it meditation, call it talking to yourself if you like, but if it's positive it can provide very effective support and reinforcement to the treatment program you're on.

I reckon everyone, deep down, in a crisis has a Something they turn to, even if they don't know what to call it. A committed atheist may say with total sincerity, "I believe in *nothing at all!*" In that case I guess the equation means that when they're really in trouble, *nothing at all* will help or sustain them.

Like all of the various treatment options I've mentioned, the key is finding out what works for you. What feels right. Only you know that.

Simply put: if you tell yourself a treatment isn't going to work for you then it won't. If you're going to try something, really give it a try.

6.12 Giving up has consequences too

There is another option to trying different therapies, alternative approaches or one more type of medication. You can quit.

> **"Most men don't fear death. They fear those things – the knife, the shipwreck, the illness, the bomb – which precede, by microseconds if you're lucky and many years if you're not, the moment of death."**
>
> *- Terry Pratchett*
> British author, Alzheimer's fighter and 'assisted death' campaigner

Accept your fate. Die. Let your health fail or even accelerate the process. I've known blokes who've done exactly that. Hell, I was nearly one of them. Some days I think I'm still vulnerable to the idea.

In 2013 over 25 Australian blokes per 100,000 aged between 40 and 44 committed suicide. Between ages 45 and 54 it was just under 24 per 100,000. (By comparison less than 9.5 women per 100,000 died by their own hand in those age bands.) All up, 1885 Aussie blokes topped themselves that year, compared to 637 women. That's nearly seven per day, and that average is pretty steady from 2009 to 2013. It doesn't include things like 'accidental' overdoses, stacking the car, or alcohol poisoning – it's just death by 'known' deliberate action.

I have to tell you, in every case I've ever known, whether the death has been by active assistance or passive giving in to the body's breakdown, the pain has been felt by those left behind.

Even blokes who'd convinced themselves that nobody cared were mourned. Family, friends – people who "wish they could have done something". Often added to that phrase: "if only I'd known…"

I recently read an interview with the widow of a bloke who'd topped himself, possibly because of trouble at work. Maybe. She wasn't sure.

"You're like a fish flapping around in no water. That's the thing with suicide. They do it and you never have those answers. I will never know why. It was so well-hidden."

Those people then have to live with their pain, and their guilt, however misplaced you think that may be. If you've kept your pain, your unwellness, your depression a secret, whether it's from embarrassment or the thought that they couldn't help anyway, then your death is a shock they weren't prepared for. If you've kept quiet out of concern about 'upsetting' them, may I just point out how *really* upset they'll be when you die!

Every suicide directly affects at least six other people. Those people are family, friends, co-workers, medical staff, counsellors. Suicide doesn't have just one victim.

Yes, you're going to die anyway. We all are. I could finish writing this book and be hit by a bus. But that doesn't mean we can't try to make the most of the life we've got, or that we should underestimate what that life might mean to others.

It's your decision. But please don't rush into it. Have you really tried everything? Have you really spoken to everyone and anyone who might help? Are you ready and willing to actually say, "Goodbye" to people? Because that's a luxury that suicides have that's denied to accident victims and those who die suddenly.

It's your life. If you're well enough to be reading this then it's your responsibility. Please take that responsibility seriously.

Simply put: Dying is one way to resolve the physical and psychological pain of ageing, but you should remember that it can cause a lot of pain and distress to those left behind.

6.13 Measuring success – honestly

How much help any doctor or therapist can be depends on two things really.

One is how much you're prepared to tell them about how you're feeling. You (and only you) can control that. But if you want someone to fight on your behalf, it makes sense to give them all the ammunition that you can, doesn't it?

The other thing is beyond your control, and that's their own personal belief about 'change of life' in blokes. You'll get a feel for that when you're talking to them.

If it feels like they don't believe you, or dismiss the idea of a 'mid-life crisis' as either non-existent or a bit of a joke, then I reckon you ought to go talk to someone else.

For one thing, there's a lot of evidence that there is something going on. In 2013 researchers at the Northwestern Memorial Hospital estimated that in the USA over 5 million men were affected by recognisable male menopausal symptoms.

You're not alone, okay?

Simply put: if you don't think the person you're talking to is taking your concerns seriously, then get a second opinion. It's your body, your brain. If you're being honest with yourself, then you know if there's something wrong.

How do you know if whatever approach you're taking is working? Sometimes it's obvious, if you've got a really chronic symptom that clears up within days of taking your new tablet or starting your new exercise or whatever.

Sometimes the benefits are slower or more subtle – harder to pick.

Here's a tip:

- at the very start, before you begin the series of treatments or therapy or course of tablets, write down a list of *all* of the aches, pains and symptoms that are bothering you;
- make four columns beside the list of symptoms;
- in the first column, before you've started doing anything different, grade each symptom on a scale of 1 to 10 as to how much it bothers or affects you, write the date at the top of the column, then put the list away somewhere safe;
- after a month do the same grading in the second column, then put it away again;
- after two, then three months, repeat the process using the third and fourth columns of the list;
- then have a good look at all of the ratings, and compare the results.

If you can recognise an improvement, then great! It's working, whatever "it" is. You're getting healthier, maybe without even noticing.

If there's no improvement, or worse still a decline (or a bunch of nasty new symptoms you want to add to the list) then it's time to look at another option.

Like I said, it's all about finding what works best for **you**.

(If that all sounds too complicated, I've knocked together a form you can use. It's at the back of this book – you can copy it, or go to this page of my website and print it for yourself:

If you've got some other technique of your own then, of course, use it. The point is to monitor your own health and healing, in whatever way is easiest and most effective for you. Not to do so can be downright dangerous.

Think of it as like driving along a busy road. Even if it's a road you know well, maybe you drive along it every day, it's still important to keep your eyes on what's going on. Murphy's Law says that the time you don't will be the time someone slams on their brakes in front of you, or tears out of a side street, or there are unexpected roadworks. And remember, the worst thing about Murphy's Law is that Murphy was an optimist.

> "Keep your eyes on the road and your hands upon the wheel!"
> *- Jim Morrison (the Doors)*
> 'Roadhouse Blues'

Simply put: whatever treatments or therapies you try, you are the best person to decide whether or not they're working for you – so take responsibility for your own health.

.o0o.

7 NOW <u>DO</u> SOMETHING...

Menopause is as real for men as it is for women. It's different, and it's different for every individual bloke, but hormone production in the male body does change with time. And that change in your body's chemistry leads to other changes, which in turn can be made worse or better by choices you make and the way you live your life.

The "mid-life crisis" can hit any man. Sometimes the pressures of work, family, and the world in general can get on top of you. The changes your body is going through with age may make it even harder to cope with them – that can be when the *crisis* hits. It can affect the way you feel and the way you think. But it doesn't have to ruin your life, and it certainly doesn't have to end it.

Maybe you're looking in the mirror and not liking what you see. Maybe you can't do some of the fun things you used to. Maybe the past looks rosier than it did at the time, and a whole lot rosier than the present or future.

All of those are things you can do something about. It won't necessarily be easy, although you might be pleasantly surprised at how readily some changes can happen. But there are a lot of options available to you. It's never too late, or too early, to improve the quality of your own life.

"It always seems impossible, until it's done!"
- Nelson Mandela
South African statesman

There are things you can do to maintain your physical, mental and psychological health day by day, or improve it if it's not all you want it to be. There are interventions - treatments and therapies that can also help. Some might seem obvious even if you've been, for whatever reason, reluctant to approach them. Others you might think are unconventional, but they've got their supporters who swear by them. You don't know what works for you until you try.

But the best start is being honest with yourself. Being honest with your family should help too, and especially with your doctor/therapist/treatment provider.

> **"Your health and your body are a reflection of how you live your life. The decisions you make can influence that positively or negatively. Poor decisions can take ten years or more off your healthspan."**
> *- Dr. Brian Dixon*
> Executive Director Health Science & Education, USANA

I like how Dr. Dixon distinguishes between lifespan and "healthspan". The difference between how long you spend on the planet, and how long you're in a reasonable condition to enjoy it.

Exactly what that means is up to you. You know how physically and mentally active you want to be. You might want to still be running or cycling for an hour or more per day when you're in your eighties. You may be content by that age if you can walk from your armchair to the mailbox and back without wheezing, as long as you can still finish all the crosswords and puzzles in the daily newspaper.

I'm not here to push you in a direction that I want you to go. I want to support you in finding your own destination and reaching it.

But to do that you have to make a move.

What matters most is that if there's a problem you

- recognise it

- admit it

- do something about it.

Reading this book is a good start – it might just give you some ideas. Talking to someone is good, too.

Set goals for yourself. Make them achievable, and figure out a roadmap for getting there. Don't just say, "I'm gonna get healthy!" or even, "I'm gonna shed 50 kilos in a year!" Give yourself measurable targets – milestones. If you make them too big or difficult or scary, it's really hard to maintain momentum, or even enthusiasm.

"By the yard it's hard – by the inch it's a cinch!"

Think about how much and why your health matters to you.

I really hope you're not saying, "I have to stay alive and healthy for my family – they need me."

If they *need* you, you're not doing it right. You're seeing them, raising them even, as reliant on you. You haven't equipped them to be independent. Financially, or more importantly, in their heads.

The cemeteries are full of healthy people. Accidents happen. Bad stuff happens to good people. If you care about your family make sure they don't need you – make sure they *want* you. Be healthy enough, alive enough, to spend real, good time with them. Not at work, not in the gym. With *them*. Don't let the changes your body is going through get in the way of that.

Now: don't just sit there thinking, 'Yes, I must do something.'

DO it!

Go on-line. Check the phone book. Walk down the main street looking at shopfronts. However you do it, **find** someone who's working in a field that you trust or want to explore. **Talk** to them.

Tell them what your problem is and accept their **help**.

Then don't expect them to do it all for you. Be **actively involved**.

It's your body, your health, your life. Your responsibility.

GO AND BE THE BEST THAT YOU CAN BE.

REFERENCES

Chapter 2

www.Biology.stackexchange.com *Circatrigintan cycle of salivary testosterone in human male* Celec et al. (2003) Biological Rhythm Research 34: 305-315.

www.huffingtonpost.com *The Truth About Menopause For Men* Ryan Buxton, 4/3/2015

www.mydr.com.au *What is male menopause?* February 2013

www.wichitapaincenter.com *Male hormones and their function* 2015

Raymond. G. Burnett M.D. *Menopause – All Your Questions Answered* Contemporary Books, 1987

Willard L. Koukkari and Robert B. Sothern *INTRODUCING BIOLOGICAL RHYTHMS - A Primer on the Temporal Organization of Life* Springer, 2006

Derek Llewellyn-Jones *Every Man* Oxford University Press, 1991

Jill Margo *Man Maintenance* Penguin, 1996

Dr. Peter O'Connor *Understanding the Mid-Life Crisis* Sun, 1990

Christian Nordqvist *Male Menopause* Medical News Today, September 2013

Matty Silver *Do Men Get Menopause?* Sydney Morning Herald, 27/5/2014

Chapter 3

www.DiabetesAustralia.com.au *Understanding Diabetes* updated 19/12/2013

www.emedicinehealth.com *Osteoporosis* William C. Shiel Jr., MD, FACP, FACR

www.healthline.com *Rhinophyma* Anna Giorgi, medically reviewed by George Krucik, MD, 17/9/2012

www.LTMensclinic.com *Low Testosterone Promotes Abdominal Obesity in Ageing Men* 10/6/2014

www.mayoclinic.org *Erectile Dysfunction* Mayo Clinic Staff 2014

www.MedicineNet.com *Hot flushes* December 2014

www.ncbi.nlm.nih.gov *Testosterone for the ageing male; current evidence and recommended practice* Roger D Stanworth and T Hugh Jones March 2008 www.nlm.nih.gov *Aging changes in the male reproductive system* US National Library of Medicine (Medline Plus)

www.Sexualhealth.com *Ejaculation and orgasm* David Sobel, MD JD, September 2011

www.skincarephysicians.com *Causes of Ageing Skin* American Academy of Dermatologists, 2010

www.spineuniverse.com *Osteopenia and Osteoporosis* 21/3/2014

www.webmd.com/healthy-ageing *Sarcopenia with Ageing* Article reviewed by William Blahd M.D. on 3/8/2014

Will Brink *Preventing Sarcopenia* in Life Extension Magazine, January 2007

Jack Challoner *Amazing Body Facts and Trivia* New Burlington, 2011

Bridget A. English (editor) *Your Brain: A User's Guide* National Geographic, 2012

D.A. Gray & J. Woulfe *Lipofuscin and Aging: A Matter of Toxic Waste* Scientific Aging Knowledge Environment, 2005

Regina Hamlin M.D., John McDonald Ph.D. and Glen Putnam *The Science of Sense* UNIttogether, 2009

Derek Llewellyn-Jones *Every Man* Oxford University Press, 3rd Edition 1991

Dr. David Perlmutter MD *Grain Brain* Yellow Kite, 2014

Farid Saad, Antonio Aversa, Andrea M Isidori and Louis J Gooren *Testosterone as Potential Effective Therapy in Treatment of Obesity in Men with Testosterone Deficiency: A Review* in Current Diabetes Reviews, March 2012

Dawn Stover (editor) *Secrets of Staying Young – The science of healthy aging* Scientific American, 2015

Chapter 4

www.qz.com *Our Poor Sleeping Habits Could Be Filling Our Brains With Neurotoxins* Vivian Giang, 10/6/2015

www.qz.com *I Once Tried To Cheat Sleep And For A Year I Succeeded* Akshat Rathi, 18/6/2015

www.sciencedaily.com *Addiction & addictive behaviours* 15/8/2011

www.yournewswire.com *Depression is an Allergic Reaction to Inflammation, Research Suggests* Tim de Chant 2015

Dr. Peter Brown (editor) *Health Care of the Older Adult* Woodslane, 2010

Brian Kaplan MBBCh *When Men Reach A Certain Age...* Health & Homeopathy, Spring 2003

Marty Klein *Sex Addiction: A Dangerous Clinical Concept* SIECUS
  Report, June – July 2003
Derek Llewellyn-Jones *Every Man* Oxford University Press, 3rd Edition
  1991
Dr. Derek Milne *Coping With A Mid-life Crisis* NHS On-line, February
  2014

Paul Azinger quoted in *A Good Walk Spoiled* by John Feinstein, Little,
  Brown and Company, 1995
Chris Walker cited in '*From The Depths Of Despair*' by Peter Badel, The
  Sunday Mail, 28/6/2015
Personal comment – Chris Benoit, Melbourne 1994

Chapter 5

www.chopra.com/ccl/neuroscience-insight *How to Break Bad Habits* Dr.
  Sarah McKay, January 2016
www.health.howstuffworks.com/wellness *How does alcohol make you
  drunk?* Laurie L. Dove, 5/9/2014
www.Healthyeating.sfgate.com *Can We Live Without Salt Consumption?*
  Sharon Perkins
www.heart.org *About Cholesterol* American Heart Association, 21/4/2014
www.mayoclinic.org *Erectile Dysfunction* Mayo Clinic Staff, 2014
www.medicalnewstoday.com *What Is Salt?* Christian Nordqvist,
  14/11/2013
www.who.int/tobacco/mpower/2009/en *World Health Organisation Report
  on the Global Tobacco Epidemic 2009*

Bridget A. English (editor) *Nature's Best Remedies* National Geographic,
  2015
Lyle MacWilliam, MSc, FP *NutriSearch Comparative Guide to Nutritional
  Supplements* 5th Consumer Edition for Australia & New Zealand, Northern
  Dimensions Publishing, 2014
Dr. Libby Weaver *The Calorie Fallacy* Little Green Frog, 2014
Paleo for Beginners Rockridge Press, 2013
Steps lower early death risk in Sydney Morning Herald, 6/11/2015
Smoking and risk behaviours in Australia, 2007-8 Australian Bureau of
  Statistics 'At a glance...' series
Tobacco Smoking in Australia, 2007-08 Australian Bureau of Statistics 'At a
  glance...' series
Worried about your memory? Here's what you can do... Brochure by
  Alzheimer's Australia, 2013

Chapter 6

www.betterhealth.vic.gov.au *The effect of lower testosterone levels with increasing age* Andrology Australia, January 2014

www.medicalqigong.com.au *The Difference Between Medical Qigong and Health Qigong* Dr. Bernard Shannon, November 2015

www.mytherapist.co *The Difference Between Chinese & Shiatsu Massage* Jessica Brown, September 2015

www.naturaltherapypages.com.au *Massage Therapy – Shiatsu*

www.sciencedaily.com *Older age does not cause testosterone levels to decline in healthy men* The Endocrine Society, 7/6/2011

www.WebMD.com *What Is Homeopathy?* Medical reference from Healthwise 14/11/2014

Mr. Cooper Ali-Shabazz *Warrior Mysticism: The Acquisition of Power* Self-published, 2015

R. H. Fletcher & K. M. Fairfield *Vitamins for Chronic Disease Prevention in Adults: Clinical Applications* Journal of the American Medical Association, 2002

Antoniette Gomez *Chakra Mindset* Exhale, 2014

Dharma Singh Khalsa & Cameron Stauth *Meditation as Medicine* Atria, 2009

Lyle MacWilliam, MSc, FP *NutriSearch Comparative Guide to Nutritional Supplements* 5th Consumer Edition for Australia & New Zealand, Northern Dimensions Publishing, 2014

Dr. Brian Morton *Why Men Should See Their GP* Wellness & Heart Health, Summer 2010

Roy Moynihan *Diagnosis excessive* The Saturday Paper, 3-9/10/2015

Peter Munro *Hard Times – Tradies' breakdown and suicide in Australia* Sydney Morning Herald 'Good Weekend', 5/3/2016

Erin O'Reilly, Marika Sevigny, Kelley-Anne Sabarre & Karen P. Phillips *Perspectives of Complementary & Alternative Medicine Practitioners in the Support and Treatment of Infertility* University of Ottawa, September 2014

Johnny Pink *The True Value of Martial Arts* Self-published, 2014

Catherine Zuckerman *How Milk Goes Down Around The World* National Geographic, May 2015

Andre Borschberg article *Record Breaker* by Emma Howard, Guardian Weekly, 10/7/2015

Causes of Death, Australia 2013 Australian Bureau of Statistics On-line issue 31/3/2015

Andrew McLachlan quoted in *Medical Mythbuster* – Sydney Alumni Magazine, University of Sydney, Semester One, 2015

Personal comment – Warren Hirst, Ballina, 2015
Personal comment – Peter Lecke, Vanuatu, 2016
Personal comment – Dr. Gerard Lewis, Brisbane, 2014
Personal comment – Dr. Armonia Rodriguez Marin, Baja California, 2015
Personal comment - Dr. Bill Meyers, Landsborough, 2016
Personal comment – Celia Roberts BSc, Brisbane, 2015
Personal comment – Yu Yan, Stratford-Upon-Avon, 2014

.o0o.

BONUS #1: Renoir's Top 6 Tips for surviving mid-life:

HONESTY.

First and foremost, be honest with yourself about how you're feeling – physically and emotionally. Then it's easier to be honest with your family, and with the doctor or therapist who you want to help you.

EAT WELL.

As often as possible, choose good food. Support your diet with good quality supplements. (If you want to know what I take go to www. meredian.usana.com)

ACTIVITY.

Don't just sit around watching yourself get old. Exercise regularly. It doesn't have to be super-strenuous, but get some deep breaths going and get your heart rate up – not all the time, but regularly.

RELAX.

Don't try to be 'on' all the time. Take time out to do stuff that calms you down and puts a smile on your face. Sleep when you're tired.

SKIN CARE.

Taking proper care of the outside helps to protect and strengthen what goes on inside. (You can check out what I use at the website above.)

EVALUATE.

Whatever therapy or routine you try, keep a regular record of what shape you're in. That's the best way of recognizing what works for you.

Remember, whatever your concerns or problems, you're not alone. There are solutions, and there is support. So keep the undertaker at bay – make sure that *you* drive the **HEARSE**!

BONUS # 2: Evaluation – Is this treatment working?

HOW DO I FEEL?

It's important that you test how well a treatment or therapy is working for you. This process, including this form, can help you to do that.

List all your aches, pains and symptoms, and rate how bad they feel **before** you start the program of treatment or therapy. Note the date on that top row.

A month later, as the treatment continues, rate how each of those things now feel. Don't think about how they were – rate how they *are* _now_ at the time you're writing. Add any new problems to the list.

Do it again a month later, then again three months after the Start date. Can you see a real improvement? If "Yes" then stick with it! If "No" – it's time to try something else.

Here's an example, then there's a blank form you can copy and use. (You can also find it at https://menshealthaquietword.com/ evaluation-is-this-treatment-working/)

	SYMPTOMS		SEVERITY		

	START 3/7	+1 month	+2 mths	+3 mths
Daily headaches	8	7	4	2
Dizzy spells	9	7	4	2
Constipation	4	6	6	6
Short temper	7	6	5	3
Stomach cramps			4	4

In this example, you can see a clear improvement in some symptoms, which is great. But it looks like the treatment's having a bad effect on this bloke's digestion. If he explains that to his doctor they can work out a way to fix it. Maybe a new pill, or a change in dosage, or a change in diet if the doctor reckons the original treatment may be reacting with particular foods.

SYMPTOMS

SEVERITY
on scale 1 (mild) – 10 (terrible)

	START Date:	+1 month	+2 mths	+3 mths

BONUS # 3: Some useful resources

What I use for nutrition supplements and skin care:

Troubled by depression:

In Australia

www.beyondblue.org.au - phone 1300 224636

\- phone 13 11 14
www.lifeline.org.au/Get-Help/Online-Services/crisis-chat

In the US

\- phone (212) 673 -3000
www.samaritansnyc.org/24-hour-crisis-hotline
NDMDA Depression hotline – phone 800-826-3632

In the UK

www.depressionuk.org

www.samaritans.org
- phone 0845 790 9090

Looking for the company and support of other blokes?

In Australia – the Australian Mens Shed Association

– www.mensshed.org

or email

- amsa@mensshed.net

Get a comprehensive, confidential health assessment

Thanks...

There are, of course, many people who I'd like to thank.

For inspiration -
- My beloved Meredith.
- The late Spike Milligan.
- The late Sir Terry Pratchett.
- Matt & Patrick Walker.
- Dr. Myron Wentz.

For support and advice, technical or otherwise -
- Mr. Cooper Ali-Shabazz,
- Prof. Darrell Crawford,
- Pam Ferry,
- Angus Gardner,
- Dr. Doug Gray,
- Warren Hirst,
- Robert Lodge,
- Dr. Hamish Lunn,
- Dr. Bill Meyers,
- Iain Moore,
- Dr. Angus Thomson,
- Celia Roberts,
- Alastair Wallace,
- Maggie Wildblood,
- Yu Yan & Paige Du

Finally, and especially, all of you who bought and/or are reading this. I sincerely hope it helps!

Renoir

Printed in Australia
AUOC02n1330101116
280391AU00002B/28/P

9 780994 617484